WEIGHT LOSS FOR MEN

FINALLY FIT
AGAIN

*The Ultimate Men's Health Book To
Lose Weight With Complete Meal
Plans, Workout Plans, Intermittent
Fasting, Keto Diet, Healthy Meal Prep*

BRYANT EVANS

Table of Contents

PART I

Introduction

The world of strength training is growing increasingly chaotic and downloading this book is the first step you can take towards getting a little bit more clarity about it. The first step is also always the easiest, however, which is why the information you find in the following chapters is so important to take to heart as they are not concepts that can be put into action immediately. If you file them away for when they are really needed in the gym, however, then when the time comes to use them, you will be glad you did learn them. What I have discovered after years of strength training, in fact, is that most people think that there is not a theoretical aspect of the exercises they are performing. Instead, knowing it is extremely important to acquire a better form.

To that end, the following chapters will discuss the primary preparedness principals that you will need to consider if you ever hope to realistically be ready to build up your strength over a period of time. Only by having the right knowledge you will be able to lay out a clear plan to get bigger, leaner and stronger.

In this book, you will then learn everything you need to know about strength training and how to take your gains to the next level. The same principles have helped me and other hundreds of people to get the body they desired.

There are plenty of books on this subject on the market, thanks again for choosing this one! Every effort was made to ensure it is full of as much useful information as possible, please enjoy!

Chapter 1: 5 Reasons why most people fail to get bigger

Are you training hard but cannot increase your muscle mass? Read this chapter on the 5 reasons why you are not increasing your muscle mass: you will probably discover that you are making one of these big mistakes. Do not worry, though: understanding the problem is the first step towards solving it.

1. Do you eat enough?

The problem could be easy to solve, do you eat enough? When you embark on a journey into fitness it is can happen to get caught up in exercising and skip on the nutritional aspect. I'm sure you know that 'abs are made in the kitchen'; well, it could not be truer. Eating enough calories (and good ones) is the first step towards getting leaner.

To increase your muscle mass, you have to eat the right amount of the right food, including carbohydrates, proteins, and fats. Your body uses the food you eat to build new muscle tissue after you destroyed the old one in training. In order to do that, it is important to consume enough protein.

Some of the best sources of protein are:

- Chicken

- Fish

- Turkey

- Lean minced meat

- eggs

- meat, broccoli, salmon

Other sources of protein

- Milk flakes

- Greek yogurt

- Quark cheese

- Beans and legumes

- Nuts

A high-protein diet is fundamental to build muscles. Experts and pro bodybuilders have stated, over the years, that consuming 1.2 – 2.0g of protein per kg of weight is a good ratio to keep building lean muscle mass over time. If you are not able to get this amount trough diet alone than food supplements can come hand.

2. Do you train hard enough?

If you have been training for a while, but have not made some gains, it could be due to a lack of training. Do you train hard enough? Our body reacts quickly under pressure and if you're not increasing weights over time, then you could run into a stall zone. So do not settle!

Your body is not made to change itself and it is your duty to give it the right stimulus so that it can actually grow. If you want to get faster results, add more intensity to your training.

3. Rest and recovery

Rest is a fundamental aspect when it comes to any fitness routine. Your muscles require rest to grow stronger and that is the reason why so many athletes choose a training routine divided into days. For example, one day they train legs and the day after the arms, making sure that every part of the body receives at least one day of rest (try to train every muscle group at least once a week).

Even sleeping is very important: when we sleep deeply our bodies repair muscle fibres. It is recommended to sleep 8 hours per night, although my advice is to sleep more if you can.

4. Do you drink too much alcohol?

Drinking too much alcohol can destroy muscle growth. Alcohol does not contain valuable nutrients but has many calories, 7 per gram to be precise. As a result, it is easy to "drink your calories" without even thinking about it. If you are on a fitness regimen of any kind, it is advisable to avoid alcohol consumption. However, a drink has never killed anybody, just be reasonable.

5. Are you over-training?

Training with high frequency and intensity activates muscle growth. Therefore, it is fundamental to train different days during the week: 4 days of weight training and 1-2 of aerobic activity is advisable. If you begin a program, complete it! Too many times athletes give up or say that a certain workout does not work "for them" (as if this could be a thing), but the key is constancy. It may take a while to see results, do not give up!

Many bodybuilders, like Arnold, have mentioned the famous 'mind and body connection', so try to keep your attention on the muscle you are training while you do the exercises. It is also a question of 'sensations' and how your muscles contract and expand.

Instead of simply doing the training, focus on the exercise and visualize the growth you are generating.

Chapter 2: 10 Rules to increase your muscle mass

It is always challenging to give the 10 rules of anything. However, when it comes to growing muscles, it is important to have some guidance. This is why we give you 10 rules to increase your lean muscle mass for a more defined body.

1. Give space to recovery: it is not true that more is better, especially for the frequency. It is true that you can train only 1 muscle a day and then before you go back to training that muscle should pass 6/8 days, but the organs of "disposal" are always the same and run the risk of overloading. You can make short periods with high frequency, but these must then have periods of supercompensation.

2. You should sleep very well: it is not only the quantity (7/9 hours per night) but the quality of sleep. An excellent component of deep sleep, it is the basic element for recovery and growth. Sleep must be mainly nocturnal, it is well known by those who work for shifts that daytime sleep has different qualities.

3. Eat often: at least 6 times, breakfast, mid-morning, lunch, afternoon, dinner and after dinner; and in any case, use the rule of about 2.5 hours between one meal and another. If you spend many hours between lunch and dinner, introduce two snacks in the afternoon.

4. Eat a balanced diet: with every meal, give space to all the nutrients. Not only proteins and carbohydrates, fats are also great allies, since are hormonal mediators, provide calories and improve recovery.

5. Do not train too long: do not spend too much time working on your endurance, since it does more harm than good to muscle's growth.

6. Think positive: the mind is a great ally for the optimization of metabolic

processes; Positivity helps the hormonal systems to overcome the negativity generated by the inevitable obstacles and setbacks of everyday life. It is essential to define the goals (even in the short term) to go to the gym with clear ideas already, aware that you will have an excellent training session.

7. Rely on basic movements: squats, deadlifts, bench, lunges, are the fundamentals; mass is not built by abusing side wings, crosses or arms. Dedicate yourself to these exercises by changing sets, repetitions and recovery times. Then there may be periods in which the complementary serve to unload the joints and give a different kind of intensity.

8. Do not just focus on some muscle groups: first, you have to build a solid foundation, do not do like those beginners who already after 6 months want to focus only on one or two muscles.

9. Use the right supplements: pay attention, do not abuse them, simply select the main ones; good proteins, BCAAs (branched amino acids) or a pool of amino acids, glutamine, creatine, a support for your joints, HMB. These are already more than enough to support and integrate a diet that must follow the correct guidelines.

10. Choose a motivating gym: well-equipped but with what you really need, lots of dumbbells and barbells, benches and maybe 2 racks for the squat. Usually, in these environments, you can also find training partners to share workouts, goals and discussions. Training in a sterile and "losing" environment is certainly not very motivating and does not establish the spirit necessary to achieve the goals.

The points to be developed would still be many but in reality, with the 10 you have read you are already well on your way to get bigger and leaner. Success is built from the basics, especially when you are just starting out.

Chapter 3: How to actually build lean muscles

It is difficult to build muscle mass, but with constancy you can do it; however, if you want to develop it quickly, you can find some compromises, like accept to gain some fat along with muscle mass and stop some other type of training, such as running, so that the body starts to focus on developing muscles. You also need to eat more by using the right strategies and doing those physical activities that allow you to increase your muscles. Here are some of the key steps to build lean muscles for real.

1. Start with a basic strength training. Most of the exercises that involve the main muscle groups start with a strength training that activates more joints and that allows you to lift a whole greater weight, such as bench presses for the pectorals, those behind the head for the deltoids, the rower with a barbell for the back and the squats for the legs. They are all exercises that allow you to lift heavier weights while still remaining active and keeping enough energy to better stimulate muscle growth.

2. Engaged thoroughly. The key to developing muscle mass is to do high intensity exercises; with a light exercise, even if protracted in time, the muscles almost never find the right conditions for decomposition and then rebuild. Schedule sessions for 30-45 minutes 3-4 times a week (every other day); it may seem like an easily manageable schedule but remember that during each session you have to engage as intensely as possible. Initially, the muscles may be sore, but over time the routine will become easier.

3. During each training session, only lift the weights that you are able to support by assuming the correct posture. Test your limits to find the right ballast you can lift, doing different repetitions with different dumbbells.

You should be able to do 3-4 sets of 8-12 repetitions without feeling the need to put them on the ground; if you are not able, reduce the weights. In general, 6-12 repetitions stimulate the growth of the volume of the muscles, while fewer repetitions favour the increase of the strength at the expense of the size of the same. If you can do 10 or more repetitions without experiencing a burning sensation, you can increase the weight; remember that you do not increase muscle mass until you challenge yourself to the limit.

4. Lift weights explosively. Raise the handlebars quickly but lower them slowly.

5. Keep the correct posture. To develop a precise technique, you have to do each repetition in the right way; beginners must commit to doing only the repetitions that they are able to perform based on the level of resistance. Find your rhythm for each exercise; you do not have to reach muscle failure when you're at the beginning. You should be able to complete the whole movement without getting to bend down or change position; if you cannot, switch to less heavy dumbbells. In most cases, it starts with the arms or legs extended. During the first sets, you should work with a personal trainer who will teach you the correct posture of the various exercises before continuing alone.

6. Toggle the muscle groups. You do not have to keep the same group moving at every set, otherwise, you may get to damage your muscles, so be sure to alternate, so every time you train you can work intensely for an hour on a different muscle group. If you do physical activity three times a week, try doing the exercises as follows:

First session: do exercises for the chest, triceps and biceps;

Second session: concentrate on the legs;

Third session: do abs and chest

7. Be careful not to reach a stall level. If you always do the same exercise repeatedly, you cannot get improvements; you have to increase the weight of the barbell and when you reach a plateau even with this, change exercise. Be aware of progress and see if your muscles do not seem to change, because it may be a sign that you need to make changes in your physical activity routine.

8. Rest between one workout and another. For those who have a rapid metabolism, the rest period is almost as important as the exercise itself. The body needs time to regenerate muscle mass without burning too many calories by doing other activities. Running and other cardio exercises can effectively prevent muscle growth; then take a break between the different sessions. Sleep well at night, so that you feel

regenerated for the next session.

9. Create a mind/muscle connection. Some research has found that it can optimize results in the gym. Instead of focusing on your day or the girl next to you, committed to developing a muscle-oriented mindset that helps you achieve your goals. Here's how:

Every time you complete a repetition, visualize the muscle growth you wish to achieve.

If you are lifting with one hand, place the other on the muscle you wish to develop; in this way, you should perceive exactly which muscle fibres are working and you can stay focused on the effort.

Remember that the amount of weight on the bar is not as important as you may think, but it is the effect that weight has on the muscle that allows you to get the volume and strength you are looking for; this process is closely related to the mentality and the goal of your concentration.

10. Eat whole foods rich in calories. You should get the calories from nutritious whole foods, so you have the right energy to quickly accumulate muscle mass. Those rich in sugar, white flour, trans fats and added flavours contain many calories but few nutrients and increase the fat instead of developing the muscle. If you want to develop the muscles and their definition, you have to opt for a wide variety of whole foods that are part of all the food groups.

11. Eat protein rich in calories, like steak and roast beef, roast chicken (with skin and dark meat), salmon, eggs and pork; proteins are essential when you want to increase muscle mass. Avoid bacon, sausages and other sausages, because they contain additives that are not suitable if you eat it in large quantities.

12. Consume lots of fruit and vegetables of all kinds; these foods provide the essential fiber and nutrients, as well as keeping you well hydrated.

13. Do not neglect whole grains, such as oatmeal, whole wheat, buckwheat and quinoa; avoid white bread, biscuits, muffins, pancakes, waffles and other similar foods.

14. Add legumes and nuts, such as black beans, Pinto, Lima, walnuts, pecans, peanuts and almonds to your diet.

15. Eat more than you think you need. Eat when you're hungry and stop when you feel satisfied? This may seem completely normal, but when you're trying to gain muscle mass quickly, you have to eat more than usual. Add another portion to each meal or even more if you can handle it; the body needs the energy to develop the muscles: it is a simple concept.

To this end, a good breakfast includes a cup of oatmeal, four eggs, two or more slices of grilled ham, an apple, an orange and a banana.

For lunch, you can eat a wholemeal sandwich with chicken, several handfuls of dried fruit, two avocados and a large salad of cabbage and tomatoes.

For dinner, you can consider a large steak or some other source of protein, potatoes, vegetables and double the portions of each dish.

16. Eat at least five meals a day. You must not wait to be hungry before eating again; you have to constantly replenish your body when you are trying to develop muscle mass. It will not be this way forever, so take advantage and enjoy the moment! Eat two more meals in addition to the traditional three (breakfast, lunch and dinner).

17. Take supplements, but do not solely on them. You do not have to think

that protein shakes do all the work for you; for your purpose, you need to get the most calories from high-calorie whole foods; Having said that, you can definitely speed up the process by taking certain supplements that have not proven to be harmful to the body.

Creatine is a protein supplement that can increase muscle; usually, it is sold as a powder that is dissolved in water and drunk a few times a day.

Protein shakes are fine when you cannot get enough calories through normal meals.

18. Keep yourself hydrated. Training hard to gain muscle mass can quickly dehydrate you. To cope with this risk, always carry a bottle of water with you wherever you go and drink whenever you are thirsty; in theory, you should drink about 3 litres of fluids a day, but you should drink more, especially before and after training.

Avoid sugary or carbonated drinks, because they do not help your overall fitness and may even take you back when you do strength exercises.

Alcohol is also harmful for your purpose: it dehydrates and leaves a feeling of exhaustion.

19. Try to get to know your body better. Do you know which foods are effective for you and which are not? During this phase of change, pay attention to what happens to your muscles. Each person is different and the food that is not suitable for one person can instead be very useful for another; if you do not notice improvements within a week, make changes and try something else the following week.

20. Sleep more than what you think you should. Sleep is essential to allow muscles to develop; try to sleep at least seven hours a night, although the

ideal would be 8-9 hours.

21. Focus only on strength training. You may like to do cardio exercises (sports like running and so on), but these activities require a further effort of the body (muscles and joints) and consume the energy you need to build muscle mass. In general, cardio activities should be included in an exercise routine for general health and well-being, but if you are currently struggling to increase muscle volume quickly, you need to focus on this for a few months, so you can reach your goal.

Chapter 4: Tips to keep making gains

- Always ask a friend for help when doing the most difficult lifting exercises, such as bench press; these are high risk movements and it is always important to have some support to be able to do more repetitions.

- Keep motivation high. Find a friend who's training with you, sign up for a weightlifting fan forum or keep a diary to monitor progress; whatever you choose, the important thing is that you inspire yourself.

- If you currently do not have dumbbells and you've never done weight lifting so far, start with push-ups and chin-ups, which are quite challenging for a beginner.

- Make the push-ups easier: start from the normal position of the push-ups and lower the body very slowly; go down as far as possible without touching the floor with your chest and abs. Later, relieved after resting your knees on the ground and start again. This is an excellent solution when you are not yet strong enough to be able to do traditional push-ups.

- Make sure you stay focused. Take breaks only when you need them and not when you feel tired; it is only in this way that you can develop psychological endurance.

Chapter 5: Example of a training schedule

The frequency of this hypothetical schedule for mass training, provides 4 days of training per week, with about 10-12 repetitions per exercise.

The mass program is a middle ground between heavy weights / high intensity training and volume/pump training. You work on strength, hypertrophy, rotating muscle definition and progression, accustoming the body to weight and intensity of work with a growing load plan, which reaches your ideal combination for mass growth.

It is essential, in fact, to know your body and your own ceilings, to prepare and act upon a successful program.

Weekly training schedule (Monday - Friday)

Chest and abs

Legs

Rest

Shoulders - triceps

Back - biceps

Daily mass gym program

1st day - chest and abs

crossed exercises with dumbbells - flat bench

distances with barbell - flat bench

multipower inclined (or with dumbbells)

cross exercises with cables

crunches (3 sets - 15 repetitions)

abs with elbows in support and knees on the chest (3 sets - 15 repetitions)

2nd Day - legs

45-degree press

squat with barbell

standing calf (3 sets - 15 repetitions)

seated calf (3 sets - 15 repetitions)

leg extension

leg curl

3rd Day - shoulders and deltoids

slow forward exercise with barbell - seated

pull at the bottom with a barbell

lateral raises with dumbbells

push down

French press around the neck with a barbell

bench presses

4th Day - back

pull ups

pullover

pulley

deadlift

curl with dumbbells

curl reverse socket with a barbell

Recovery between the series should be carried out for about 1 minute and a half (1 '30).

The first month these exercises should be performed with at least 3 sets and about 10-12 repetitions, with non-high loads. In case you are not trained enough, you can think of sets of 12-10-8 repetitions, where you start with 12 and perform 8 repetitions in the third set.

The second month you can go up to 4 sets with 10 repetitions or 12 if the body keeps up with the pace. It will not be easy to get to the twelfth repetition without fatigue and, in this case, you can also think about dropping with weights and get to 12 repetitions with lighter loads.

The third month you have to keep the pace but without progressing too much, with the initials 3 sets of 12 repetitions per exercise.

PART II

Smoothie Diet Recipes

The smoothie diet is all about replacing some of your meals with smoothies that are loaded with veggies and fruits. It has been found that the smoothie diet is very helpful in losing weight along with excess fat. The ingredients of the smoothies will vary, but they will focus mainly on vegetables and fruits. The best part about the smoothie diet is that there is no need to count your calorie intake and less food tracking. The diet is very low in calories and is also loaded with phytonutrients.

Apart from weight loss, there are various other benefits of the smoothie diet. It can help you to stay full for a longer time as most smoothies are rich in fiber. It can also help you to control your cravings as smoothies are full of flavor and nutrients. Whenever you feel like snacking, just prepare a smoothie, and you are good to go. Also, smoothies can aid in digestion as they are rich in important minerals and vitamins. Fruits such as mango are rich in carotenoids that can help in improving your skin quality. As the smoothie diet is mainly based on veggies and fruits, it can detoxify your body.

In this section, you will find various recipes of smoothies that you can include in your smoothie diet.

Chapter 1: Fruit Smoothies

The best way of having fruits is by making smoothies. Fruit smoothies can help you start your day with loads of nutrients so that you can remain energetic throughout the day. Here are some easy-to-make fruit smoothie recipes that you can enjoy during any time of the day.

Quick Fruit Smoothie

Total Prep & Cooking Time: Fifteen minutes

Yields: Four servings

Nutrition Facts: Calories: 115.2 | Protein: 1.2g | Carbs: 27.2g | Fat: 0.5g | Fiber: 3.6g

Ingredients

- One cup of strawberries
- One banana (cut in chunks)
- Two peaches
- Two cups of ice
- One cup of orange and mango juice

Method:

1. Add banana, strawberries, and peaches in a blender.

2. Blend until frothy and smooth.

3. Add the orange and mango juice and blend again. Add ice for adjusting the consistency and blend for two minutes.

4. Divide the smoothie in glasses and serve with mango chunks from the top.

Triple Threat Smoothie

Total Prep & Cooking Time: Ten minutes

Yields: Four servings

Nutrition Facts: Calories: 132.2 | Protein: 3.4g | Carbs: 27.6g | Fat: 1.3g | Fiber: 2.7g

Ingredients

- One kiwi (sliced)
- One banana (chopped)
- One cup of each
  - Ice cubes
  - Strawberries
- Half cup of blueberries
- One-third cup of orange juice
- Eight ounces of peach yogurt

Method:

1. Add kiwi, strawberries, and bananas in a food processor.

2. Blend until smooth.

3. Add the blueberries along with orange juice. Blend again for two minutes.

4. Add peach yogurt and ice cubes. Give it a pulse.

5. Pour the prepared smoothie in smoothie glasses and serve with blueberry chunks from the top.

Tropical Smoothie

Total Prep & Cooking Time: Fifteen minutes

Yields: Two servings

Nutrition Facts: Calories: 127.3 | Protein: 1.6g | Carbs: 30.5g | Fat: 0.7g | Fiber: 4.2g

Ingredients

- One mango (seeded)
- One papaya (cubed)
- Half cup of strawberries
- One-third cup of orange juice
- Five ice cubes

Method:

1. Add mango, strawberries, and papaya in a blender. Blend the ingredients until smooth.

2. Add ice cubes and orange juice for adjusting the consistency.

3. Blend again.

4. Serve with strawberry chunks from the top.

Fruit and Mint Smoothie

Total Prep & Cooking Time: Fifteen minutes

Yields: Two servings

Nutrition Facts: Calories: 90.3 | Protein: 0.7g | Carbs: 21.4g | Fat: 0.4g | Fiber: 2.5g

Ingredients

- One-fourth cup of each
  - Applesauce (unsweetened)
  - Red grapes (seedless, frozen)
- One tbsp. of lime juice
- Three strawberries (frozen)
- One cup of pineapple cubes
- Three mint leaves

Method:

1. Add grapes, lime juice, and applesauce in a blender. Blend the ingredients until frothy and smooth.

2. Add pineapple cubes, mint leaves, and frozen strawberries in the blender. Pulse the ingredients for a few times until the pineapple and strawberries are crushed.

3. Serve with mint leaves from the top.

Banana Smoothie

Total Prep & Cooking Time: Ten minutes

Yields: Four servings

Nutrition Facts: Calories: 122.6 | Protein: 1.3g | Carbs: 34.6g | Fat: 0.4g | Fiber: 2.2g

Ingredients

- Three bananas (sliced)
- One cup of fresh pineapple juice
- One tbsp. of honey
- Eight cubes of ice

Method:

1. Combine the bananas and pineapple juice in a blender.

2. Blend until smooth.

3. Add ice cubes along with honey.

4. Blend for two minutes.

5. Serve immediately.

Dragon Fruit Smoothie

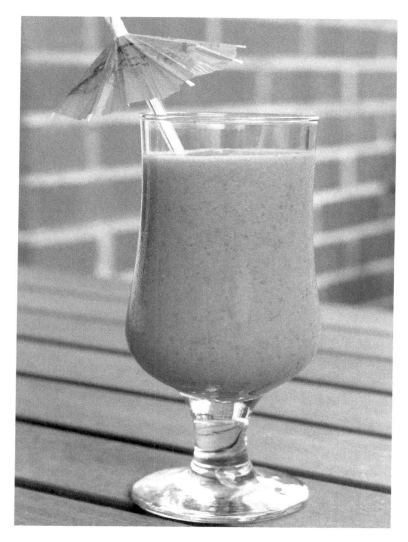

Total Prep & Cooking Time: Twenty minutes

Yields: Four servings

Nutrition Facts: Calories: 147.6 | Protein: 5.2g | Carbs: 21.4g | Fat: 6.4g | Fiber: 2.9g

Ingredients

- One-fourth cup of almonds
- Two tbsps. of shredded coconut
- One tsp. of chocolate chips
- One cup of yogurt
- One dragon fruit (chopped)
- Half cup of pineapple cubes
- One tbsp. of honey

Method:

1. Add almonds, dragon fruit, coconut, and chocolate chips in a high power blender. Blend until smooth.

2. Add yogurt, pineapple, and honey. Blend well.

3. Serve with chunks of dragon fruit from the top.

Kefir Blueberry Smoothie

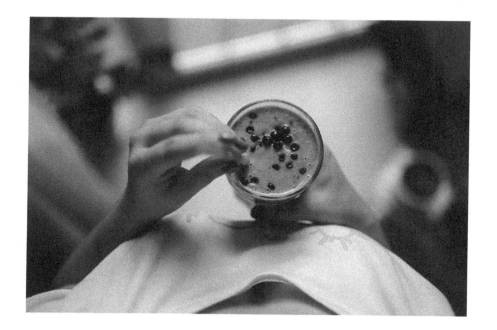

Total Prep & Cooking Time: Fifteen minutes

Yields: Two servings

Nutrition Facts: Calories: 304.2 | Protein: 7.3g | Carbs: 41.3g | Fat: 13.2g | Fiber: 4.6g

Ingredients

- Half cup of kefir
- One cup of blueberries (frozen)
- Half banana (cubed)

- One tbsp. of almond butter
- Two tsps. of honey

Method:

1. Add blueberries, banana cubes, and kefir in a blender.

2. Blend until smooth.

3. Add honey and almond butter.

4. Pulse the smoothie for a few times.

5. Serve immediately.

Ginger Fruit Smoothie

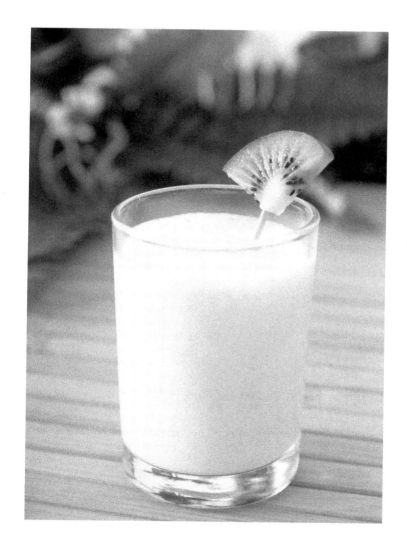

Total Prep & Cooking Time: Fifteen minutes

Yields: Two servings

Nutrition Facts: Calories: 160.2 | Protein: 1.9g | Carbs: 41.3g | Fat: 0.7g | Fiber: 5.6g

Ingredients

- One-fourth cup of each
  - o Blueberries (frozen)
  - o Green grapes (seedless)
- Half cup of green apple (chopped)
- One cup of water
- Three strawberries
- One piece of ginger
- One tbsp. of agave nectar

Method:

1. Add blueberries, grapes, and water in a blender. Blend the ingredients.

2. Add green apple, strawberries, agave nectar, and ginger. Blend for making thick slushy.

3. Serve immediately.

Fruit Batido

Total Prep & Cooking Time: Fifteen minutes

Yields: Six servings

Nutrition Facts: Calories: 129.3 | Protein: 4.2g | Carbs: 17.6g | Fat: 4.6g | Fiber: 0.6g

Ingredients

- One can of evaporated milk
- One cup of papaya (chopped)
- One-fourth cup of white sugar
- One tsp. of vanilla extract
- One tsp. of cinnamon (ground)
- One tray of ice cubes

Method:

1. Add papaya, white sugar, cinnamon, and vanilla extract in a food processor. Blend the ingredients until smooth.

2. Add milk and ice cubes. Blend for making slushy.

3. Serve immediately.

Banana Peanut Butter Smoothie

Total Prep & Cooking Time: Ten minutes

Yields: Four servings

Nutrition Facts: Calories: 332 | Protein: 13.2g | Carbs: 35.3g | Fat: 17.8g | Fiber: 3.9g

Ingredients

- Two bananas (cubed)
- Two cups of milk
- Half cup of peanut butter
- Two tbsps. of honey
- Two cups of ice cubes

Method:

1. Add banana cubes and peanut butter in a blender. Blend for making a smooth paste.

2. Add milk, ice cubes, and honey. Blend the ingredients until smooth.

3. Serve with banana chunks from the top.

Chapter 2: Breakfast Smoothies

Smoothie forms an essential part of breakfast in the smoothie diet plan. Here are some breakfast smoothie recipes for you that can be included in your daily breakfast plan.

Berry Banana Smoothie

Total Prep & Cooking Time: Twenty minutes

Yields: Two servings

Nutrition Facts: Calories: 330 | Protein: 6.7g | Carbs: 56.3g | Fat: 13.2g | Fiber: 5.5g

Ingredients

- One cup of each
  - Strawberries
  - Peaches (cubed)
  - Apples (cubed)
- One banana (cubed)
- Two cups of vanilla ice cream
- Half cup of ice cubes
- One-third cup of milk

Method:

1. Place strawberries, peaches, banana, and apples in a blender. Pulse the ingredients.

2. Add milk, ice cream, and ice cubes. Blend the smoothie until frothy and smooth.

3. Serve with a scoop of ice cream from the top.

Berry Surprise

Total Prep & Cooking Time: Ten minutes

Yields: Two servings

Nutrition Facts: Calories: 164.2 | Protein: 1.2g | Carbs: 40.2g | Fat: 0.4g | Fiber: 4.8g

Ingredients

- One cup of strawberries
- Half cup of pineapple cubes
- One-third cup of raspberries
- Two tbsps. of limeade concentrate (frozen)

Method:

1. Combine pineapple cubes, strawberries, and raspberries in a food processor. Blend the ingredients until smooth.

2. Add the frozen limeade and blend again.

3. Divide the smoothie in glasses and serve immediately.

Coconut Matcha Smoothie

Total Prep & Cooking Time: Twenty minutes

Yields: Two servings

Nutrition Facts: Calories: 362 | Protein: 7.2g | Carbs: 70.1g | Fat: 8.7g | Fiber: 12.1g

Ingredients

- One large banana
- One cup of frozen mango cubes
- Two leaves of kale (torn)
- Three tbsps. of white beans (drained)
- Two tbsps. of shredded coconut (unsweetened)
- Half tsp. of matcha green tea (powder)
- Half cup of water

Method:

1. Add cubes of mango, banana, white beans, and kale in a blender. Blend all the ingredients until frothy and smooth.

2. Add shredded coconut, white beans, water, and green tea powder. Blend for thirty seconds.

3. Serve with shredded coconut from the top.

Cantaloupe Frenzy

Total Prep & Cooking Time: Ten minutes

Yields: Three servings

Nutrition Facts: Calories: 108.3 | Protein: 1.6g | Carbs: 26.2g | Fat: 0.2g | Fiber: 1.6g

Ingredients

- One cantaloupe (seeded, chopped)
- Three tbsps. of white sugar
- Two cups of ice cubes

Method:

1. Place the chopped cantaloupe along with white sugar in a blender. Puree the mixture.

2. Add cubes of ice and blend again.

3. Pour the smoothie in serving glasses. Serve immediately.

Berry Lemon Smoothie

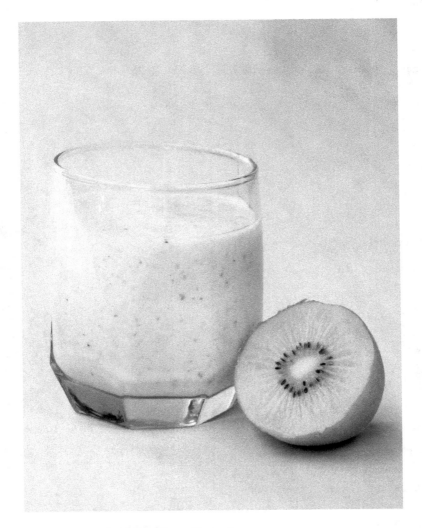

Total Prep & Cooking Time: Ten minutes

Yields: Four servings

Nutrition Facts: Calories: 97.2 | Protein: 5.4g | Carbs: 19.4g | Fat: 0.4g | Fiber: 1.8g

Ingredients

- Eight ounces of blueberry yogurt
- One and a half cup of milk (skim)
- One cup of ice cubes
- Half cup of blueberries
- One-third cup of strawberries
- One tsp. of lemonade mix

Method:

1. Add blueberry yogurt, skim milk, blueberries, and strawberries in a food processor. Blend the ingredients until smooth.

2. Add lemonade mix and ice cubes. Pulse the mixture for making a creamy and smooth smoothie.

3. Divide the smoothie in glasses and serve.

Orange Glorious

Total Prep & Cooking Time: Ten minutes

Yields: Four servings

Nutrition Facts: Calories: 212 | Protein: 3.4g | Carbs: 47.3g | Fat: 1.5g | Fiber: 0.5g

Ingredients

- Six ounces of orange juice concentrate (frozen)
- One cup of each
  - Water
  - Milk
- Half cup of white sugar
- Twelve ice cubes
- One tsp. of vanilla extract

Method:

1. Combine orange juice concentrate, white sugar, milk, and water in a blender.

2. Add vanilla extract and ice cubes. Blend the mixture until smooth.

3. Pour the smoothie in glasses and enjoy!

Grapefruit Smoothie

Total Prep & Cooking Time: Ten minutes

Yields: Two servings

Nutrition Facts: Calories: 200.3 | Protein: 4.7g | Carbs: 46.3g | Fat: 1.2g | Fiber: 7.6g

Ingredients

- Three grapefruits (peeled)
- One cup of water
- Three ounces of spinach
- Six ice cubes
- Half-inch piece of ginger
- One tsp. of flax seeds

Method:

1. Combine spinach, grapefruit, and ginger in a high power blender. Blend until smooth.

2. Add water, flax seeds, and ice cubes. Blend smooth.

3. Pour the smoothie in glasses and serve.

Sour Smoothie

Total Prep & Cooking Time: Ten minutes

Yields: Two servings

Nutrition Facts: Calories: 102.6 | Protein: 2.3g | Carbs: 30.2g | Fat: 0.7g | Fiber: 7.9g

Ingredients

- One cup of ice cubes
- Two fruit limes (peeled)
- One orange (peeled)
- One lemon (peeled)
- One kiwi (peeled)
- One tsp. of honey

Method:

1. Add fruit limes, lemon, orange, and kiwi in a food processor. Blend until frothy and smooth.

2. Add cubes of ice and honey. Pulse the ingredients.

3. Divide the smoothie in glasses and enjoy!

Ginger Orange Smoothie

Total Prep & Cooking Time: Ten minutes

Yields: One serving

Nutrition Facts: Calories: 115.6 | Protein: 2.2g | Carbs: 27.6g | Fat: 1.3g | Fiber: 5.7g

Ingredients

- One large orange
- Two carrots (peeled, cut in chunks)
- Half cup of each
    - Red grapes
    - Ice cubes
- One-fourth cup of water
- One-inch piece of ginger

Method:

1. Combine carrots, grapes, and orange in a high power blender. Blend until frothy and smooth.

2. Add ice cubes, ginger, and water. Blend the ingredients for thirty seconds.

3. Serve immediately.

Cranberry Smoothie

Total Prep & Cooking Time: One hour and ten minutes

Yields: Two servings

Nutrition Facts: Calories: 155.9| Protein: 2.2g | Carbs: 33.8g | Fat: 1.6g | Fiber: 5.2g

Ingredients

- One cup of almond milk
- Half cup of mixed berries (frozen)
- One-third cup of cranberries
- One banana

Method:

1. Blend mixed berries, banana, and cranberries in a high power food processor. Blend until smooth.

2. Add almond milk and blend again for twenty seconds.

3. Refrigerate the prepared smoothie for one hour.

4. Serve chilled.

Creamsicle Smoothie

Total Prep & Cooking Time: Ten minutes

Yields: Two servings

Nutrition Facts: Calories: 121.3 | Protein: 4.7g | Carbs: 19.8g | Fat: 2.5g | Fiber: 0.3g

Ingredients

- One cup of orange juice
- One and a half cup of crushed ice
- Half cup of milk
- One tsp. of white sugar

Method:

1. Blend milk, orange juice, white sugar, and ice in a high power blender.

2. Keep blending until there is no large chunk of ice. Try to keep the consistency of slushy.

3. Serve immediately.

Sunshine Smoothie

Total Prep & Cooking Time: Thirty minutes

Yields: Four servings

Nutrition Facts: Calories: 176.8 | Protein: 4.2g | Carbs: 39.9g | Fat: 1.3g | Fiber: 3.9g

Ingredients

- Two nectarines (pitted, quartered)
- One banana (cut in chunks)
- One orange (peeled, quartered)
- One cup of vanilla yogurt
- One-third cup of orange juice
- One tbsp. of honey

Method:

1. Add banana chunks, nectarines, and orange in a blender. Blender for two minutes.

2. Add vanilla yogurt, honey, and orange juice. Blend the ingredients until frothy and smooth.

3. Pour the smoothie in glasses and serve.

Chapter 3: Vegetable Smoothies

Apart from fruit smoothies, vegetable smoothies can also provide you with essential nutrients. In fact, vegetable smoothies are tasty as well. So, here are some vegetable smoothie recipes for you.

Mango Kale Berry Smoothie

Total Prep & Cooking Time: Ten minutes

Yields: Four servings

Nutrition Facts: Calories: 117.3 | Protein: 3.1g | Carbs: 22.6g | Fat: 3.6g | Fiber: 6.2g

Ingredients

- One cup of orange juice
- One-third cup of kale
- One and a half cup of mixed berries (frozen)
- Half cup of mango chunks
- One-fourth cup of water
- Two tbsps. of chia seeds

Method:

1. Take a high power blender and add kale, orange juice, berries, mango chunks, chia seeds, and half a cup of water.

2. Blend the ingredients on high settings until smooth.

3. In case the smoothie is very thick, you can adjust the consistency by adding more water.

4. Pour the smoothie in glasses and serve.

Breakfast Pink Smoothie

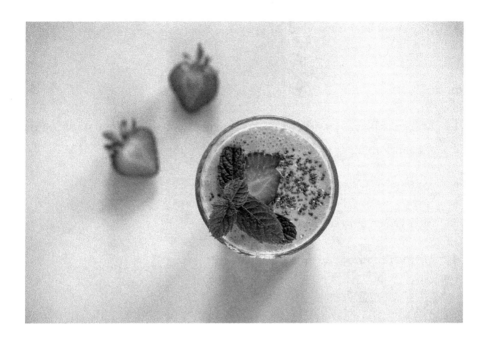

Total Prep & Cooking Time: Ten minutes

Yields: Two servings

Nutrition Facts: Calories: 198.3 | Protein: 12.3g | Carbs: 6.3g | Fat: 4.5g | Fiber: 8.8g

Ingredients

- One and a half cup of strawberries (frozen)
- One cup of raspberries
- One orange (peeled)

- Two carrots
- Two cups of coconut milk (light)
- One small beet (quartered)

Method:

1. Add strawberries, raspberries, and orange in a blender. Blend until frothy and smooth.

2. Add beet, carrots, and coconut milk.

3. Blend again for one minute.

4. Divide the smoothie in glasses and serve.

Butternut Squash Smoothie

Total Prep & Cooking Time: Five minutes

Yields: Four servings

Nutrition Facts: Calories: 127.3 | Protein: 2.3g | Carbs: 32.1g | Fat: 1.2g | Fiber: 0.6g

Ingredients

- Two cups of almond milk
- One-fourth cup of nut butter (of your choice)
- One cup of water
- One and a half cup of butternut squash (frozen)
- Two ripe bananas
- One tsp. of cinnamon (ground)
- Two tbsps. of hemp protein
- Half cup of strawberries
- One tbsp. of chia seeds
- Half tbsp. of bee pollen

Method:

1. Add butternut squash, bananas, strawberries, and almond milk in a blender. Blend until frothy and smooth.

2. Add water, nut butter, cinnamon, hemp protein, chia seeds, and bee pollen. Blend the ingredients f0r two minutes.

3. Divide the smoothie in glasses and enjoy!

Zucchini and Wild Blueberry Smoothie

Total Prep & Cooking Time: Ten minutes

Yields: Three servings

Nutrition Facts: Calories: 190.2 | Protein: 7.3g | Carbs: 27.6g | Fat: 8.1g | Fiber: 5.7g

Ingredients

- One banana
- One cup of wild blueberries (frozen)
- One-fourth cup of peas (frozen)
- Half cup of zucchini (frozen, chopped)
- One tbsp. of each
  - Hemp hearts
  - Chia seeds
  - Bee pollen
- One-third cup of almond milk
- Two tbsps. of nut butter (of your choice)
- Ten cubes of ice

Method:

1. Add blueberries, banana, peas, and zucchini in a high power blender. Blend the ingredients for two minutes.

2. Add chia seeds, hemp hearts, almond milk, bee pollen, nut butter, and ice. Blend the mixture for making a thick and smooth smoothie.

3. Pour the smoothie in glasses and serve with chopped blueberries from the top.

Cauliflower and Blueberry Smoothie

Total Prep & Cooking Time: Five minutes

Yields: Two servings

Nutrition Facts: Calories: 201.9 | Protein: 7.1g | Carbs: 32.9g | Fat: 10.3g | Fiber: 4.6g

Ingredients

- One Clementine (peeled)
- Three-fourth cup of cauliflower (frozen)
- Half cup of wild blueberries (frozen)
- One cup of Greek yogurt
- One tbsp. of peanut butter
- Bunch of spinach

Method:

1. Add cauliflower, Clementine, and blueberries in a blender. Blend for one minute.

2. Add peanut butter, spinach, and yogurt. Pulse the ingredients for two minutes until smooth.

3. Divide the prepared smoothie in glasses and enjoy!

Immunity Booster Smoothie

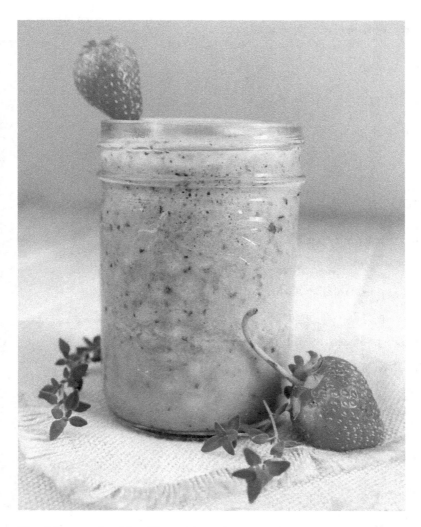

Total Prep & Cooking Time: Ten minutes

Yields: Two servings

Nutrition Facts: Calories: 301.9 | Protein: 5.4g | Carbs: 70.7g | Fat: 4.3g | Fiber: 8.9g

Ingredients

For the orange layer:

- One persimmon (quartered)
- One ripe mango (chopped)
- One lime (juiced)
- One tbsp. of nut butter (of your choice)
- Half tsp. of turmeric powder
- One pinch of cayenne pepper
- One cup of coconut milk

For the pink layer:

- One small beet (cubed)
- One cup of berries (frozen)
- One pink grapefruit (quartered)
- One-fourth cup of pomegranate juice
- Half cup of water
- Six leaves of mint
- One tsp. of honey

Method:

1. Add the ingredients for the orange layer in a blender. Blend for making a smooth liquid.

2. Pour the orange liquid evenly in serving glasses.

3. Add the pink layer ingredients in a blender. Blend for making a smooth liquid.

4. Pour the pink liquid slowly over the orange layer.

5. Pour in such a way so that both layers can be differentiated.

6. Serve immediately.

Ginger, Carrot, and Turmeric Smoothie

Total Prep & Cooking Time: Forty minutes

Yields: Two servings

Nutrition Facts: Calories: 140 | Protein: 2.6g | Carbs: 30.2g | Fat: 2.2g | Fiber: 5.6g

Ingredients

For carrot juice:

- Two cups of water
- Two and a half cups of carrots

For smoothie:

- One ripe banana (sliced)
- One cup of pineapple (frozen, cubed)
- Half tbsp. of ginger
- One-fourth tsp. of turmeric (ground)
- Half cup of carrot juice
- One tbsp. of lemon juice
- One-third cup of almond milk

Method:

1. Add water and carrots in a high power blender. Blend on high settings for making smooth juice.

2. Take a dish towel and strain the juice over a bowl. Squeeze the towel for taking out most of the juice.

3. Add the ingredients for the smoothie in a blender and blend until frothy and creamy.

4. Add carrot juice and blend again.

5. Pour the smoothie in glasses and serve.

Romaine Mango Smoothie

Total Prep & Cooking Time: Five minutes

Yields: Two servings

Nutrition Facts: Calories: 117.3 | Protein: 2.6g | Carbs: 30.2g | Fat: 0.9g | Fiber: 4.2g

Ingredients

- Sixteen ounces of coconut water
- Two mangoes (pitted)
- One head of romaine (chopped)
- One banana
- One orange (peeled)
- Two cups of ice

Method:

1. Add mango, romaine, orange, and banana in a high power blender. Blend the ingredients until frothy and smooth.

2. Add coconut water and ice cubes. Blend for one minute.

3. Pour the prepared smoothie in glasses and serve.

Fig Zucchini Smoothie

Total Prep & Cooking Time: Ten minutes

Yields: Two servings

Nutrition Facts: Calories: 243.3 | Protein: 14.4g | Carbs: 74.3g | Fat: 27.6g | Fiber: 9.3g

Ingredients

- Half cup of cashew nuts
- One tsp. of cinnamon (ground)
- Two figs (halved)
- One banana
- Half tsp. of ginger (minced)
- One-third tsp. of honey
- One-fourth cup of ice cubes
- One pinch of salt
- Two tsps. of vanilla extract
- Three-fourth cup of water
- One cup of zucchini (chopped)

Method:

1. Add all the listed ingredients in a high power blender. Blend for two minutes until creamy and smooth.

2. Pour the smoothie in serving glasses and serve.

Carrot Peach Smoothie

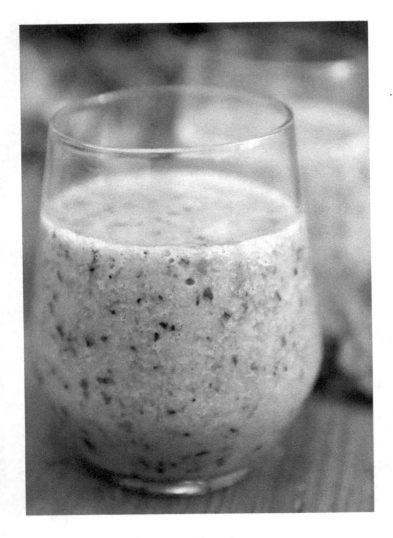

Total Prep & Cooking Time: Ten minutes

Yields: Two servings

Nutrition Facts: Calories: 191.2 | Protein: 11.2g | Carbs: 34.6g | Fat: 2.7g | Fiber: 5.4g

Ingredients

- Two cups of peach
- One cup of baby carrots
- One banana (frozen)
- Two tbsps. of Greek yogurt
- One and a half cup of coconut water
- One tbsp. of honey

Method:

1. Add peach, baby carrots, and banana in a high power blender. Blend on high settings for one minute.

2. Add Greek yogurt, honey, and coconut water. Give the mixture a whizz.

3. Pour the smoothie in glasses and serve.

Sweet Potato and Mango Smoothie
Total Prep & Cooking Time: Ten minutes

Yields: Two servings

Nutrition Facts: Calories: 133.3 | Protein: 3.6g | Carbs: 28.6g | Fat: 1.3g | Fiber: 6.2g

Ingredients

- One small sweet potato (cooked, smashed)
- Half cup of mango chunks (frozen)
- Two cups of coconut milk
- One tbsp. of chia seeds
- Two tsps. of maple syrup
- A handful of ice cubes

Method:

1. Add mango chunks and sweet potato in a high power blender. Blend until frothy and smooth.

2. Add chia seeds, coconut milk, ice cubes, and maple syrup. Blend again for one minute.

3. Divide the smoothie in glasses and serve.

Carrot Cake Smoothie

Total Prep & Cooking Time: Ten minutes

Yields: Two servings

Nutrition Facts: Calories: 289.3 | Protein: 3.6g | Carbs: 47.8g | Fat: 1.3g | Fiber: 0.6g

Ingredients

- One cup of carrots (chopped)
- One banana
- Half cup of almond milk
- One cup of Greek yogurt
- One tbsp. of maple syrup
- One tsp. of cinnamon (ground)
- One-fourth tsp. of nutmeg
- Half tsp. of ginger (ground)
- A handful of ice cubes

Method

1. Add banana, carrots, and almond milk in a blender. Blend until frothy and smooth.

2. Add yogurt, cinnamon, maple syrup, ginger, nutmeg, and ice cubes. Blend again for two minutes.

3. Divide the smoothie in serving glasses and serve.

Notes:

- You can add more ice cubes and turn the smoothie into slushy.

- You can store the leftover smoothie in the freezer for two days.

Chapter 4: Green Smoothies

Green smoothies can help in the process of detoxification as well as weight loss. Here are some easy-to-make green smoothie recipes for you.

Kale Avocado Smoothie

Total Prep & Cooking Time: Ten minutes

Yields: Two servings

Nutrition Facts: Calories: 401 | Protein: 11.2g | Carbs: 64.6g | Fat: 17.3g | Fiber: 10.2g

Ingredients

- One banana (cut in chunks)
- Half cup of blueberry yogurt
- One cup of kale (chopped)
- Half ripe avocado
- One-third cup of almond milk

Method:

1. Add blueberry, banana, avocado, and kale in a blender. Blend for making a smooth mixture.

2. Add the almond milk and blend again.

3. Divide the smoothie in glasses and serve.

Celery Pineapple Smoothie

Total Prep & Cooking Time: Ten minutes

Yields: Two servings

Nutrition Facts: Calories: 112 | Protein: 2.3g | Carbs: 3.6g | Fat: 1.2g | Fiber: 3.9g

Ingredients

- Three celery stalks (chopped)
- One cup of cubed pineapple
- One banana
- One pear
- Half cup of almond milk
- One tsp. of honey

Method:

1. Add celery stalks, pear, banana, and cubes of pineapple in a food processor. Blend until frothy and smooth.

2. Add honey and almond milk. Blend for two minutes.

3. Pour the smoothie in serving glasses and enjoy!

Cucumber Mango and Lime Smoothie

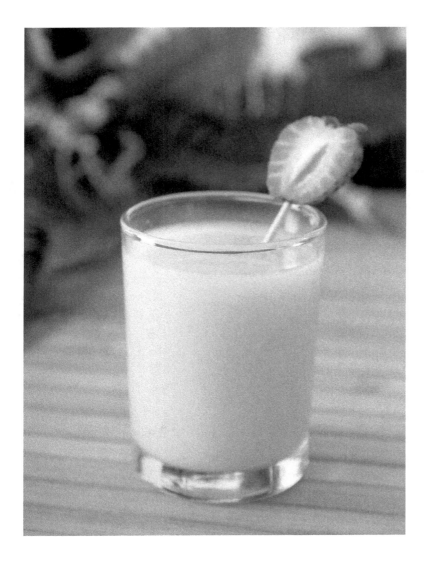

Total Prep & Cooking Time: Ten minutes

Yields: Two servings

Nutrition Facts: Calories: 165 | Protein: 2.2g | Carbs: 32.5g | Fat: 4.2g | Fiber: 3.7g

Ingredients

- One cup of ripe mango (frozen, cubed)
- Six cubes of ice
- Half cup of baby spinach leaves
- Two leaves of mint
- Two tsps. of lime juice
- Half cucumber (chopped)
- Three-fourth cup of coconut milk
- One-eighth tsp. of cayenne pepper

Method:

1. Add mango cubes, spinach leaves, and cucumber in a high power blender. Blend until frothy and smooth.

2. Add mint leaves, lime juice, coconut milk, cayenne pepper, and ice cubes. Process the ingredients until smooth.

3. Pour the smoothie in glasses and serve.

Kale, Melon, and Broccoli Smoothie

Total Prep & Cooking Time: Ten minutes

Yields: One serving

Nutrition Facts: Calories: 96.3 | Protein: 2.3g | Carbs: 24.3g | Fat: 1.2g | Fiber: 2.6g

Ingredients

- Eight ounces of honeydew melon
- One handful of kale
- Two ounces of broccoli florets
- One cup of coconut water
- Two sprigs of mint
- Two dates
- Half cup of lime juice
- Eight cubes of ice

Method:

1. Add kale, melon, and broccoli in a food processor. Whizz the ingredients for blending.

2. Add mint leaves and coconut water. Blend again.

3. Add lime juice, dates, and ice cubes. Blend the ingredients until smooth and creamy.

4. Pour the smoothie in a smoothie glass. Enjoy!

Kiwi Spinach Smoothie

Total Prep & Cooking Time: Ten minutes

Yields: Two servings

Nutrition Facts: Calories: 102 | Protein: 3.6g | Carbs: 21.3g | Fat: 2.2g | Fiber: 3.1g

Ingredients

- One kiwi (cut in chunks)
- One banana (cut in chunks)
- One cup of spinach leaves
- Three-fourth cup of almond milk
- One tbsp. of chia seeds
- Four cubes of ice

Method:

1. Add banana, kiwi, and spinach leaves in a blender. Blend the ingredients until smooth.

2. Add chia seeds, ice cubes, and almond milk. Blend again for one minute.

3. Pour the smoothie in serving glasses and serve.

Avocado Smoothie

Total Prep & Cooking Time: Ten minutes

Yields: Two servings

Nutrition Facts: Calories: 345 | Protein: 9.1g | Carbs: 47.8g | Fat: 16.9g | Fiber: 6.7g

Ingredients

- One ripe avocado (halved, pitted)
- One cup of milk
- Half cup of vanilla yogurt
- Eight cubes of ice
- Three tbsps. of honey

Method:

1. Add avocado, vanilla yogurt, and milk in a blender. Blend the ingredients until frothy and smooth.

2. Add honey and ice cubes. Blend the ingredients for making a smooth mixture.

3. Serve immediately.

PART III

WHAT IS METABOLISM?

Metabolism is typically used when we are describing different chemical reactions that help to maintain healthy organisms and cells. There are two types of metabolism:

- Anabolism: the synthesis of the compounds that the cell need.

- Catabolism: the breaking down of the molecules to get energy.

Metabolism is closely linked to a person's nutrition and how they use their available nutrients. Bioenergetics tells us how our metabolic or biochemical paths for our cells use energy. Forming energy is a vital component in metabolism.

Good nutrition is the key to metabolism. Metabolism requires nutrients so they can break down to produce energy. This energy is needed to make new nucleic acids, proteins, etc.

Diets need nutrients like sulfur, phosphorus, nitrogen, oxygen, hydrogen, carbon, and 20 other inorganic elements. These elements are received from proteins, lipids, and carbohydrates. Water, minerals, and vitamins are necessary.

Your body gets carbs in three different ways from food: sugar, cellulose, and starch. Sugars and starches form essential sources of energy for us humans.

Body tissues need glucose for everyday activities. Sugars and carbs give off glucose by metabolism or digestion.

Most people's diet is half carbs. These carbs typically come from macaroni, pasta, potatoes, bread, wheat, rice, etc.

The tissue builders of the body are proteins. Proteins are found in every cell of the human body. Proteins help with enzymes that carry out needed reactions, hemoglobin formation to carry the oxygen, functions, cell structure, and many other functions within the body. Proteins are needed to supply nitrogen for DNA, producing energy, and RNA genetic material.

Protein is necessary for nutrition since they have amino acids. The human body can't synthesize eight of these, and they are amino acids that are essential to us.

These amino acids are:

- Threonine

- Valine

- Phenylalanine

- Isoleucine

- Leucine

- Methionine

- Tryptophan

- Lysine

Foods that have the best quality of protein are grains, vegetables, meats, soybeans, milk, and eggs.

Fats are a more condensed form of energy. They make twice the amount of energy as proteins or carbs.

These are the functions of fats:

- Provide a reserve for energy.

- Help to absorb fat soluble vitamins.

- Forms a protection insulation and cushion around vital organs.

- Helps to form a cellular structure.

The fatty acids that are required include unsaturated acids, such as arachidonic, linolenic, and linoleic acids. These are needed in the diet. Cholesterol and saturated fats have been associated with heart disease and arteriosclerosis.

Minerals found in food don't give you energy, but they do play a role in your bodies pathways and are important regulators. There are more than 50 elements that can be found in the body. Only 25 have been deemed essential so far. Deficiency in these could produce specific symptoms.

These are the essential minerals:

- Iodine

- Fluorine

- Magnesium

- Zinc

- Manganese

- Cobalt

- Copper

- Chloride ions

- Potassium

- Sodium

- Iron

- Phosphorus

- Calcium

Vitamins are known as organic compounds that the human body is unable to synthesize by itself, so they need to be found within your diet. These are the most important vitamins in metabolism:

- Pantothenic Acid

- Nicotinic acid or Niacin

- B2 or riboflavin

- Vitamin A

Metabolism's chemical reactions are grouped within your metabolic pathways.

This gives the chemicals that come from your nutrition to be changed through several different steps along with another chemical. This is done with a series of enzymes.

Enzymes are important for your metabolism because they give organisms the ability to achieve the reactions that they need for energy. These also work along with the others that release energy. Enzymes are basically catalysts that let these reactions happen efficiently and quickly.

PHASE 1

While on this diet you will rotate the way you eat between three phases:

- Phase One – Monday and Tuesday:

- Phase Two – Wednesday and Thursday:

- Phase Three – Friday, Saturday, and Sunday:

- Repeat this for four weeks.

Every phase focuses on different healthy, whole foods to help reduce your liver stress, calm your adrenal glands, and feed your thyroid. Now, let's look at phase one and some recipes to get you started.

Phase One – low-fat, moderate-protein, high-glycemic

One of the main things that phase one will help you with is by regulating your adrenal glands. The adrenal glands secrete stress hormones, which is only useful when you are in immediate danger. When you aren't in danger, all it will do for you is raise your cortisol level, which causes weight gain.

In phase one, you will eat higher glycemic fruits because they stimulate your pituitary gland, which is your pleasure center. This releases endorphins which will reduce anxiety and stress.

In phase one you will also need to do some cardio, this will help to reduce cortisol levels even more.

BREAKFAST

CINNAMON APPLE QUINOA

Serves: 2

Ingredients:

Honey

2 tsp cinnamon

2 large apples

1 ½ c water

½ c quinoa

Instructions:

Prepare the apples by coring and peeling. Chop the prepared apples into small pieces.

Place the apples, quinoa, and water into a pot. Allow the mixture to come to a boil. Place the lid on the pot and turn the heat down to a simmer. Let cook for 20 to 25 minutes. The apples should be soft, and the quinoa should have absorbed all the water.

Mix in the cinnamon and divide between two bowls.

Drizzle the top with some more cinnamon and honey.

LUNCH

MASHED CHICKPEA SALAD

Serves: 2

Ingredients:

Pepper and salt to your taste

1 ½ tbsp sunflower seeds

½ lemon, juiced

½ tsp garlic, minced

3 tbsp Dijon

2 tbsp cilantro

½ c kale, chopped

¼ c red onion, chopped

1/3 of an apple, chopped

2 celery stalks, chopped

15-oz chickpeas, rinsed and drained

1 carrot, shredded

Instructions:

Shred your carrot in a food processor and place in a large bowl.

Place the chickpeas in the processor and pulse a couple of times until well blended, but a little chunky. If you want, you can just use a potato masher.

Place chickpeas and the rest of the ingredients in the bowl with the carrot. Mix everything together and add pepper and salt to your taste.

DINNER

SLOW COOKER SPAGHETTI AND MEATBALLS

Serves: 6

Ingredients:

Meatballs:

½ tsp pepper

1 tsp salt

½ c breadcrumbs

2 eggs

1 ½ tsp oregano

¼ c parsley, minced

3 minced garlic

½ onion, grated

1 ½ lb lean ground beef

Sauce:

16-oz whole wheat spaghetti drained and cooked

4 basil leaves, sliced

14-oz crushed tomatoes

28-oz crushed tomatoes

½ tsp pepper

½ tsp salt

½ tsp sugar

4-oz tomato paste

1 tsp oregano

1 onion, chopped

3 minced garlic cloves

1 tbsp olive oil

Instructions:

Meatballs:

Your oven should be at 350. Spray a baking sheet with nonstick spray.

Mix the pepper, salt, breadcrumbs, eggs, oregano, parsley, garlic, onion, and beef together.

For the meat mixture into balls. Place them on the baking sheet, evenly spaced.

Bake until they are almost cooked, about 12 to 15 minutes. Transfer your meatballs to your slow cookers and scrape off bits of fat from the bottom of the meatballs.

Sauce:

Place the oil in a pan and heat. Place in the garlic and cook for a few seconds.

Mix in the oregano and onion. Cooking for about three minutes, the onions should be soft.

Stir in the pepper, salt, sugar, and tomato paste and cook another two minutes.

Mix in the basil and crushed tomatoes. Pour the mixture over the meatballs in your cooker.

Cook for five hours at low. Serve the mixture over your cooked spaghetti.

PHASE 2

Phase 2 – low-fat, low-carb, high-veggie, high-protein

Lean proteins provide the ingredients that create amino acids within the body. Alkaline vegetables provide enzymes and phytonutrients that break down the proteins. The amino acids are converted into muscle.

Muscles are insatiable. They need lots of fuel. The more muscle you have, the more fat you are going to burn. Muscle works for you. It burns fat that has been stored as fuel to help melt away stubborn fat. More muscle means higher metabolic rate. Muscle-building is about weight training. You can use your body weight, hand weight, weight machines, or dumbbells.

When you eat lean proteins such as chicken, fish, turkey, bison, and beef, the stomach will start to secrete pepsinogen that converts into the enzyme pepsin. This pepsin will start breaking down the protein into amino acids.

This phase isn't all about eating protein. If you were to eat nothing but protein, your body's pH balance would begin to be far too acidic and you will start to feel ill. To balance out this protein, you will be eating a lot of alkalizing vegetables like collard greens, cucumbers, spinach, kale, broccoli, and cabbage. These vegetables give the body more alkaline thus bringing the body's pH into balance.

The other good things happening in this phase is all the vitamin C that you are consuming is strengthening the adrenal glands, and we know that strong adrenal glands react less to stress.

Iodine and taurine in the vegetables will nourish the thyroid thus prepping it to release the fat-burning hormones that will be coming in the next phase.

BREAKFAST

KOREAN ROLLED OMELETTE

Serves: 1

Ingredients:

Roasted seaweed

2 pinches salt

3 eggs

½ tsp butter

Instructions:

Whisk the eggs together with some salt.

Butter a pan lightly.

Heat the pan and pour in the whisked eggs.

Let them cook until they are almost set, then place a sheet of seaweed on top.

Take a spatula and lift an edge of the egg over the seaweed. Continue to roll the egg over the seaweed. Allow it to cool slightly and then slice into one-inch pieces.

LUNCH

MARINATED TOFU WITH PEPPERS AND ONIONS

Serves: 4

Ingredients:

3 red bell peppers, seeded and sliced

1 red onion, sliced into ¼-inch thick rounds

1 tbsp honey

4 tbsp EVOO, divided

1 lb block medium tofu, sliced into ½-inch slices

Pepper and salt

¾ tsp paprika, divided

3 ½ tsp cumin, divided

¼ c garlic, minced

2/3 c lime juice

¾ c cilantro, chopped

Instructions:

Your oven should be at 450. Place foil onto a baking sheet. Mix ½ teaspoon paprika, 3 teaspoon cumin, garlic, lime juice, and ¼ cup cilantro together. Sprinkle with pepper and salt. Pour half of the marinade into a baggie. Place in the tofu. Seal the bag and shake so everything is coated. Allow to marinate at room temp for ten to fifteen minutes, flip over occasionally.

While that marinates, place the rest of the marinade in your blender. Add in honey, two tablespoons oil, and ¼ cup of cilantro. Mix until smooth, and add in pepper and salt to taste.

Mix the peppers and onion together in a bowl and season with pepper, salt, ¼ teaspoon paprika, ½ teaspoon cumin, and two tablespoons of oil.

Drain the marinade off the tofu. Sprinkle both sides with pepper and salt and place on the prepared baking sheet. Add the vegetables to the baking sheet next to the tofu.

Bake for 20 to 25 minutes, stirring the veggies a couple of times until everything is tender.

Divide the tofu and veggies among plates and top with sauce and the rest of the cilantro.

DINNER

ROAST BEEF AND VEGETABLES

Serves: 6

Ingredients:

1 lb red potatoes, halved

1 bulb fennel, thinly sliced

1 red onion, sliced

Pepper

2 tsp rosemary, chopped

Salt

2 tbsp balsamic vinegar

3 tbsp EVOO

3 lb beef rump roast, trimmed of fat

Instructions:

Your oven should be at 375. Brush the beef with a tablespoon of vinegar and oil. Then season with ½ teaspoon pepper, a teaspoon of rosemary, and two teaspoons of salt. Coat the potatoes, onion, and fennel with the rest of the salt, pepper, rosemary, vinegar, and oil. Place the veggies on the bottom of a nine by thirteen inch pan. Place the roast, fat side up, on the vegetables.

Cook until a thermometer reads 125 degrees Fahrenheit, and 1 ¼ to 1 ½ hours. Place the meat on a cutting board and rest for about ten minutes. Turn your oven up to 450. Stir the veggies and let them cook for another ten minutes. Slice the beef and serve along with the vegetables.

PHASE 3

Phase 3 – low-glycemic fruit, moderate protein, moderate carb, high healthy fat

It sounds counter-intuitive, but healthy fats from raw seeds, olive oil, avocados, and raw nuts will trigger your body to burn the dietary fat and the stored fat. You have kept your fat intake low but flooded your body with nutrients from efficient proteins, alkalizing vegetables, and whole grains. You haven't been eating fats, and your body has been burning the stored fat for energy. You might have noticed that your clothes are fitting somewhat looser, but if your body catches on, and no dietary fats are coming in, it will start to store fat again instead of burning it.

Salmon helps to promote healthy hormone balance in your adrenal and thyroid glands. Other nutrients in healthy fats will start to slow gastric emptying. This helps you feel fuller longer and stimulates the pituitary glands, and hypothalamus releases feel-good hormones and allows your body to feel satisfied and full.

BREAKFAST

BERRY COBBLER WITH QUINOA

Serves: 4

Ingredients:

1 c strawberries, frozen

2 c blackberries, frozen

¼ tsp cinnamon

¼ c almond milk

¼ c maple syrup

1 tsp vanilla

¼ c ground flaxseed

½ c coconut oil

½ c chopped walnuts

½ c quinoa flour

½ c cooked quinoa

1 c dry oats

Instructions:

Your oven should be at 375.

Mix all the ingredients together, except for the berries.

Place the berries in a nine by nine baking dish and then top with the quinoa mixture.

Cook for 35 to 40 minutes or until it has browned. You can also serve with a drizzle of honey and a dollop of Greek yogurt.

LUNCH

ITALIAN TUNA SALAD

Serves: 2

Ingredients:

¼ tsp salt

1 tbsp lemon juice

1 minced garlic clove

¼ c chopped green olives

¼ c red onion, diced

½ sweet yellow pepper, diced

3-oz black olives, sliced

½ c parsley leaves, chopped

1 c diced tomatoes

2 cans Yellowfin Tuna in Olive oil, not drained

Instructions:

Place the tuna into a bowl and break up the pieces. Mix in the rest of the ingredients. You can serve on a bun or a bed of lettuce.

DINNER

SHEET PAN STEAK AND VEGGIES

Serves: 6

Ingredients:

2 lb top sirloin

Pepper and salt

1 tsp thyme

3 minced garlic cloves

2 tbsp olive oil

16-oz broccoli florets

2 lb red potatoes

Instructions:

Your oven should be set to broil. Grease a baking sheet lightly.

Parboil the potatoes for 12 to 15 minutes and drain.

Place the broccoli and potatoes on the baking sheet. Drizzle with pepper, salt, thyme, garlic, and olive oil and toss.

Sprinkle the steak with pepper and salt and place on the baking sheet between the veggies.

Broil the steak until browned, this should take about four to five minutes on each side.

DOS AND DON'TS

Avoid these foods in all phases:

- Fat-free "diet" foods – this includes zero-cal, fat-free, or diet foods

- Artificial sweeteners

- Fruit juices and dried fruit

- Alcohol

- Caffeine – if you have to have coffee, use organic decaffeinated

- Refined sugars

- Dairy

- Corn

- Non-sprouted wheat

Phase 1:

- Meals: 3 meals and 2 fruit snacks

    o Breakfast: fruit and grain, 30 minutes after waking up

    o Fruit snack

    o Lunch: vegetable, fruit, protein, and grain

    o Fruit snack

- Dinner: vegetable, protein, and grain

- Organic when possible

- All fruits and veggies

- Protein – veggie and animal

  - Lean meat

  - Lean poultry

  - Lean fish

  - Eggs – white only

  - Beans

- Plenty or spices, herbs, broth, and condiments

- Grains

  - Sprouted and whole wheat

- Water

- No fats

Phase 2:

- Meals

  - Breakfast: veggie and protein, 30 minutes after your get up

- o Protein snack

- o Lunch: veggie and protein

- o Protein snack

- o Dinner: veggie and protein

- Low-glycemic vegetables

- Lemon and limes

- Animal protein:

  - o Lean meat

  - o Lean poultry

  - o Lean fish

  - o Shellfish

  - o Eggs- white only

- No vegetable proteins

- Condiments, spices, herbs, and broth

- No starches or grains

- No fats

- Water

Phase 3:

- Meals

  o Breakfast: veggie, grain, protein, or fat 30 minutes after waking

  o Protein, fat, or veggie snack

  o Lunch: fruit, veggie, protein, or fat

  o Protein, fat, or veggie snack

  o Dinner: starch, grain, veggie, protein, or fat

- All veggies

- Low-glycemic fruits

- Animal and veggie protein

  o Any meat

  o Liver

  o Poultry

  o Fish

  o Shellfish

  o Eggs

  o Beans

- o Seeds and nuts

- o Non-dairy proteins

- Whole starches and grains

- Condiments, spices, herbs, and broth

- Healthy fats

- Water

PART IV

Chapter One: Muscle Mass

You have probably heard by now of the many benefits of having more of your body being composed of muscle mass. And yet, I'd venture to guess you still don't know the half of it!

If you're a woman, thirty percent of your body is made up of muscle mass; for men, it's around forty. The bottom line is, we all want more muscle! Muscle gives us that long and lean appearance—with nicely shaped muscles. Muscular people are viewed as healthy people. Obviously, they are also stronger. Too much fat can lead to all kinds of health problems, not to mention all the clothes you have that you can't wear!

There are many, many reasons to desire to build more muscle, but I'll give you the one that is at the top of the list for me: muscle burns fat. That's right! Muscle burns fat not only when you're in the gym or somewhere else, hitting the weights, or doing body resistance training, it does so when you're at rest. That is correct. Muscle eats away at fat while you're lolling on the sofa watching that Sunday afternoon football game.

This is why we love muscle!

Many folks don't do weight training because they think they have to head to the gym. It's a very common myth that it's necessary to use weights in order to add muscle. But it's just that—a myth. You also don't have to purchase a room full of expensive weights, gadgets and other equipment to use to build muscle at home.

I'm going to let you in on a little secret. You can build muscle using just...you. It is true. You can use your own body's resistance against itself to burn fat and build muscle. It's awesome! This way, there are no excuses. You don't have to pay a gym membership, drive yourself there, or even leave the comfort of your own home.

I'm going to give you nine different muscle-building, fat-burning workouts, and we're going to talk—just a little—about a few things you can do in the area of diet. Yes, diet. Not "diet" as in a bad word—like "I feel miserable after eating badly for the last two weeks and I need to go on a diet." Not that sort of talk. We'll simply touch on some of the foods you should be eating and some of the food you shouldn't be if you're genuinely interested in losing some weight.

Before we get into the exercises, let's cover some basics.

How Muscle is Built

Simply put in laymen's terms, when you work out, you essentially damage your muscles. Muscle tissue is broken down. When this process happens, your body gets busy repairing and replacing these damaged tissues. To get just a little technical during this process, the body has a process on the cellular level in which it repairs or replaces the damaged muscle fibers. It fuses these fibers together to form new myofibrils (muscle protein strands). Repaired myofibrils are larger in thickness and are greater in number, thus causing muscle hypertrophy (growth). This process doesn't happen when you are lifting weights, though. It happens afterward when the body is at rest. That's why rest is absolutely a key component to muscle growth. The hard work is only half the process. But fortunately the rest—pun intended—is easy.

Chapter Two: The Upper Body

"Can we please have a moment of silence for all those stuck in traffic on the way to the gym?" —Anonymous

These aren't always the easiest exercises to do—well, actually, exercising isn't exactly easy anyway, so scratch that. The great thing about upper body work is that this is where you will begin to see results first. So, for that reason, doing upper body work can be incredibly rewarding.

1. The Classic Push-Up

Push-ups are super easy, super basic and have been around forever. The reason they've been around forever is that they're also super effective. The key is to perform them correctly. If you don't, they become wasted effort.

The proper way to do push-ups

Get on the ground, belly down. Place your palms on the floor a shoulder width apart or slightly more. Keep your body straight as you push yourself up by extending your arms. Repeat. Make sure that your arms are lifting your body weight, not the muscles on the lower half of your body. Imagine there is a plank of wood on your back starting from your head to your feet. Make sure that your body is as straight as that plank in order to maintain correct body alignment.

How many push-ups?

That depends on the kind of shape you are in when you start. When you begin to do the push-ups, do they feel easy to you? Make sure you are performing the move deliberately—not going too fast that you're using momentum. The first time you try, do as many as you can while still keeping perfect form. Afterward, for your regular sets, do two-thirds that many. So, if you did fifteen but were tired by then and beginning to lose form, use ten as a target for your sets in the beginning.

As you get stronger, make the number higher. You want to continue to be challenged. Some people do as many as one-hundred push-ups per day. Perhaps that's something you can aim for. For the average beginner, three sets of ten are reasonable.

2. Chair-Dips

This is another upper-body exercise that, while in actuality, you're using your body-weight, you'll still need a chair or a bench or something similar. When I'm out running, there's a square cement planter that has an edge to it, and it works perfectly.

Dips further work the rhomboid muscles in your back and synchronize with push-ups on working your triceps.

- Get a chair/bench or another object capable of supporting your body weight and of a similar height, as explained above. Stand with your back to it. Make sure that the object is sturdy enough to support your entire body weight. Lower yourself and place your palms on the front edge of the bench, fingers pointing forward. Tuck in your elbows to your sides. Maintain this position and walk just your feet slowly in front of you. Your body weight should be resting on your arms now. Deliberately bend your arms and lower yourself. Do this until the floor is parallel to your upper arms. If you're doing it right, you'll feel it in your back and also in your triceps. Simply hold for about a second and return to the starting position.

Do three sets. Determine the number of repetitions per set the exact same way as you did for the push-ups.

3. Diamond Push-Ups

Oh, chicken wings—and not the kind you eat. "Chicken wing" is a common term used to refer to the fat on the back of a person's upper arm as it kind of tends to sag, resulting in an unattractive "flapping in the wind" sort of scenario when you wave your arms. Nobody has time for this, people! Not when there are exercises that will blast those wings if you simply stay consistent. Almost everyone wants tight, toned arms. It's a sexy look, and it's youthful! Tight triceps can actually defy a woman's age. So don't skimp on the upper body exercises. I'm giving you three here, and all of them work your triceps, but the Diamond Push-Up works it the most of all so if you're only worried about triceps and nothing else, do this one.

- Start in the push-up position, yet instead of having your hands out to the sides, place them in front of you and put them together to create a diamond shape.
- Raise yourself until your legs are straight then lower yourself until you are two inches above the ground. You will feel the burn in those triceps. Embrace the burn! The burn means the move is working.

Choose your number of reps in the same manner with all of the upper body exercises.

Chapter Three: The Core

You must not ignore the importance of core work when it comes to resistance training. Your core muscles are the ones that essentially holds everything else together.

There's a very good chance that, no matter what you're doing, you're using your core. Having a weak core takes the power away from all the rest of your muscles. Your core muscles are also responsible for your balance and stability, which is huge. Your core is not one muscle; it's a complicated interconnected series of muscles which effectively include all of them except your arms and your legs. So, I reiterate. Working your core needs to be an incredibly important part of your exercise routine.

Think about your abs. Everybody seems to be concerned with their abdominal muscles. Many people want those six-pack muscles to show. Some just want to button their favorite jeans without lying on the bed.

There's a common misconception (still) that fat can be "spot-burned." This is simply not true. The general consensus is that fat leaves the body the same way it came on—gradually and kind of all over. Don't get me wrong on this; genetics do play a role in how our bodies store fat. Some people can be perfectly proportioned pretty much everywhere on their bodies and yet have large, unattractive bellies. Those people are still more the exception than the rule.

So, the bottom line is that you cannot target fat-burning. If you really want the fat to leave your body, there are three central areas that will require your attention: diet, cardio, and resistance training. Here we are focusing on the third, and a little later I'm going to give a quick overall snapshot of the importance of combining all three.

I'm going to give you three exercises for your core. This first one, known as a Plank, could actually be used as the only core exercise you do. It is that effective and, especially considering the other exercises you'll be doing with, will touch all the muscles in your core.

Now, remember what we said about abs and fat? Here's something many people simply don't realize. Underneath however much fat we happen to be carrying on our abdominal muscles, we all have a "six-pack." Those are muscles in each of our bodies. What people are trying to do when they say they're going for six-pack abs is burn the layers of fat that cover those muscles. As I said, and much to the sadness of myself and many others, you can't target that weight.

Additionally, I'm not going to include any kind of "sit-ups" in upper body work. They've been proven to not be as effective as other exercises that work the core muscles. Also, I personally think that unless your form is always perfect with a sit-up, you may be putting certain back muscles at risk.

4. Plank

This one is tough, but like I said, with this one exercise and all the many variations you can do with it, you can get those core muscles strong in no time.

- Start with the initial push-up position. Bend your elbows to a right angle. Let your weight rest on your forearms. You might want to get a mat or something soft to use as padding between your arms and the floor. Make sure you have a timer too. The elbows need to be beneath your shoulders directly. Your body should be forming a straight line from head to heels—like a plank. Hold this position for as long as you can without injuring yourself.

Your goal should eventually be to hold it for two minutes. I said eventually for a good reason. Planks are tough. I mean, for a lot of people, a ten-second plank and they're toast. Because so many muscles are used to hold this position, if those muscles aren't strong, it simply can't happen for very long. That's also why planks are such a good indicator of how far you've come. If, when you start it takes all you have to hold a thirty-second plank, I would venture to guess that after a religiously followed routine, within eight weeks you will have worked up to the full two minutes.

Planks are great because there are many variations of them, as well. As you get stronger, try this:

- While in plank position, lift one of your legs as high as you can and hold it there for a count of thirty. Repeat on the other side.
- You can even do a side plank. Lay down on your side with your head propped on your elbow, raise your body in that position and hold it. To increase difficulty with this one, once you are in the up position, try raising your top leg and holding it in that position.

Planks can be thought of as a "Super Move." They literally work all of your muscles. In fact, if one really wanted to, one could do planks only as their resistance training (planks in all their variations, which are many) and achieve the results they're looking for.

5. Reverse Crunch

Okay, so I realize I just got done telling you that sit-ups, which are essentially crunches, are not good for the back muscles. In fact, one physician has said that he has seen no other cause of back injury with the highest rate as traditional crunches.

However, the reverse crunch, despite its name, does not carry the same risks and is excellent at targeting your abdominal muscles.

Here's how to do it:

- Lie down on the floor and fully extend your arms and legs to the sides. Put your palms on the floor. Your arms should actually stay in one place as you perform the entire exercise.

- This is the position you will start from: your legs will be pulled up which will make your thighs form a right angle with the floor. You will want your feet together and also parallel to the floor.

- Move your legs towards your torso. At the same time, roll your pelvis backward. Raise your hips above the floor. The goal is to have your knees touching your chest.

- Hold this position for around a second, then lower back to the starting position.

Again, depending on your ability when you start, gauge the number of reps and sets by how they feel to your body and how hard it is for you to do them at first. Just make sure not to overestimate yourself too much. Muscle soreness from overdoing it is no fun!

6. Mountain Climber

Get into the top of the push-up position. This is the starting position.

- Keeping your back in a straight line, bring your right knee toward your chest. Quickly bring it back to the starting position. Do the same for the left knee. Repeat but speed up the movement, alternating legs quickly as if you were running in place with your hands on the ground.

As far as how many sets, this move isn't exactly structured that way so use seconds to guide you. Try the move until you are really struggling to continue (you'll likely be out of breath) then use two-thirds of those seconds, call it a set, and do three.

Chapter Four: The Lower Body

Working out your lower body is not to be taken lightly or skimped on when doing resistance training. One particular reason for this is because your lower body contains the largest muscle in your entire body: the gluteus maximus.

Not only do most of us like to work out this muscle because it makes us "look" better, it's also a powerhouse. This muscle, along with other gluteal muscles, is one of the great stabilizers of the human body. Keeping these muscles strong can minimize aches and pains in your lower back and hips. The muscles also give you the power you need to do simple things like walk, run, and climb.

So, whenever lower body resistance training is discussed, there are two moves that are practically givens. No, it's not because they're both somewhat torturous—it's because they are effective!

When you're doing your workout, never forget the old adage, "Pain is temporary...(fill in the blank)." Usually, people say, "pain is temporary, quitting lasts forever."

That doesn't exactly apply here, but the point is that if you aren't going to be able to tolerate a little bit of pain, you aren't going to get the same results. Workouts can hurt. Muscles burn. Sometimes by the end of a good workout, you feel like you're about to croak. As far as I'm concerned, those are the very best kind! It means you've really kicked some gluteal maximuses and made some progress for the day. You have to maintain a good attitude if you're going to embark on this journey. Results don't happen overnight, but relatively you will start to see them very quickly (although, in general people who are close to you will notice before you do.) However, nothing is more satisfying than when you do look in the mirror and see results that can't be denied, or when you put on a pair of jeans that has been an eternity since they were last wore and they button easily. It's a powerful feeling.

So, here they come, the not-always-fun but ever-so-productive lower body movements.

7. The Lunge

If you've ever done them, you're probably feeling the burn simply at the thought! When executed correctly, these babies do burn, but they are incredibly effective.

Lunges produce fast results. You will notice that your legs and derriere are more toned and attractive looking. You will feel that you're stronger and you'll notice the difference when you do cardio—assuming you do, of course.

Lunges do not require weights, although weights can be added later on to increase the difficulty as you get into better shape.

Form in lunges is very important. The same is true with all of these exercises. If you're going to put in the effort, you may as well make sure you're doing it right in order to maximize your results.

Following is how to execute a perfect lunge:

- Stand upright and keep your body straight. Pull your shoulders back and relax your chin. Keep your chin pointed forward, don't look down. Make sure the muscles in your core are tight and engaged.
- If it helps you with balance, you can use something you have on hand, like, say, a broom. Hold it crossways in front of you and let it lightly rest on your shoulders.
- Pick a leg. Step forward using that leg. Lower your hips until both your knees are forming a right angle. Make sure that your lowered knee isn't touching the floor and that your forward knee is directly above your

angle and not too far forward. Make sure that your weight is in your heels as you push yourself back up to the starting position.

- When you do push back up to the starting position, really place extra emphasis on engaging your gluteus maximus. Deliberately use the strength in that muscle to push yourself upright.

Now. Repeat. How many times? I recommend starting with three sets of ten perfectly executed lunges. If you don't feel "the burn" add a couple, or go ahead and use a barbell if you have one and put some weight on it. You can even do lunges in reverse, to vary things up.

8. Squat

Ah, the squat. If you haven't done them, you've probably heard of them if you have any friends at all who work out. Like lunges, they are simple, easy to execute, and incredibly effective at increasing muscle mask and making you stronger.

Also, like lunges, there are quite a few variations to squats that you can use as you get more fit. For now, of course, we'll focus on the simple squat. Again, form is super important.

- Stand with your feet at least shoulder-width apart. If you feel more comfortable, it's okay to place your feet a bit wider apart. As you stand, you should focus on having your weight on your heels. Extend your arms straight out. The first thing you'll do is thrust your hips back slightly as though you are about to take a seat. Then, lower yourself down like that as if you are actually about to sit down. You'll want to go as low as you can. The goal is to make your knees bent so that your legs are parallel to the floor, again almost if you were sitting in a chair. Control your knees so they don't move forward over your feet.

- The next step is simply to stand up, and when you are coming upright, squeeze your glutes at the top of the movement. So, essentially, squats are like sitting in an invisible chair, then standing up using your glutes to propel you. Very easy but super effective!

9. The Bridge

The bridge is another great one for strengthening your glutes and legs. Remember, before you even see the results of these exercises, you'll be stronger for doing them. And, if you eat right and take in enough protein (building blocks for muscle) you will increase the size of your muscle and consequently burn fat. So when you're doing these not-so-fun-at-the-time moves, keep that in mind!

- Here's how to do a bridge: Lie on the floor, flat as a pancake. Place your hands on your sides and bend your knees. Your feet should be about shoulder-width apart. Lift your hips off the floor, using your heels to push. Keep your back straight while doing this! Hold the position for a second and squeeze those glutes.
- Slowly lower back to the position you started from.

For the number of reps, use the method we discussed previously. The first time you try the exercise, go until you really feel the burn—until it's very tough to continue or until you would not be able to. However many reps that is (say it's fifteen) subtract one-third of that number and start from there.

For variety, this exercise can be performed with one leg at a time.

Chapter Five: Putting it all Together

People have different preferences in how they like to work out. To see good results from strength training, you need to work each muscle group no less than two times per week. Three times is fine and you may see faster results that way. Depending on what you want to accomplish, generally, three times is enough.

The idea is to give each muscle group a rest day in between your workouts. So people go about the entire construct differently. Some like to work their entire body in one session, then rest for a day or two and do it again, up to three times a week.

Others prefer to break the muscle group workouts up. Legs one day, arms the next, core the next, like that.

In my opinion and in consideration of the research I've done, any of the above-mentioned ways to go about it will be just as effective as another. Of course, the most important component is that it gets done.

I'd like to take a moment at the time to talk about cardiovascular workouts. I know, I know, boo, hiss. A lot of people really aren't that big on cardio. However, there's a lot to be said for a good cardio sweat session. For one thing, cardiovascular exercise improves the health of our heart and lungs. That alone should be reason enough to work some in. Also, this type of exercise, depending on the type you choose, can burn an awful lot of calories. Remember, any calories burned will contribute to that sleek, muscular look. For the muscles to come out, the fat has to come off.

Cardiovascular exercise has also been proven to affect our moods in a positive way (the same can be said for weight training.)

The best, most well-rounded exercise plans include a mixture of both. Supposing you hate cardio, you will do yourself no harm by keeping it to a minimum. The general recommendation right now is to get thirty minutes of cardio on "most" days of the week.

Given that, as an example, you could do your weights on Monday, cardio Tuesday, weights Wednesday, Cardio Thursday, weights Friday and guess what? Take the weekend off!

This is just one example of how this can all be done. You can be as creative as you want to be or as you need to be to get around a work schedule.

You could do, for instance, cardio in the morning and resistance training at night. You could work in all or part of your resistance training during your lunch hour at work.

There are no limits to the options available, so that simply means *no excuses*.

No equipment or anything fancy is required for the cardio portion either. Walking is cardio. Just walk fast enough to get your heart rate up, break a sweat and breathe a little heavy. Increase intensity as your fitness level improves.

Here's a sample plan, if you need one. I'm going to use ten reps as a standard while performing the strength training for the sake of simplicity.

Monday Morning Before Work:
Three sets of ten of each of the following:

- Push-ups
- Chair-Dips
- Diamond Push-ups

Honestly, this should take you no more than ten minutes.

Monday Lunch:

- Walk for thirty minutes

Monday Evening:

Perform three sets of the following:

- Squats
- Lunges
- Bridges
- Planks
- Mountain Climber
- Reverse Crunch

Starting out, repeat this same routine on Wednesdays and Fridays. Try this for a few weeks (or another plan of your own design) and see how it works with your schedule.

On the days that you don't walk for thirty-minutes on your lunch, per your official "schedule," do it anyway. If not that, jump on the trampoline with your little ones at night for half an hour. Ride your bike. Swim. Ski if you live near snow and/or if it's wintertime. Snow Show. Or...head to the gym. Do the elliptical or the stair-climber for half of an hour. It's really not hard to get in the minimum amount of cardio and depending on your goals, and who says you have to stop with the minimum?

If you stick to this program, you're going to see some results and you'll see them pretty quickly.

Here's another tip: throw away your scale. Okay, well you don't have to throw it away. I just don't recommend weighing yourself all the time. It could discourage you in fact, for the simple reason that muscle actually does weigh more than fat. You might gain in the beginning, and no one wants to start a workout program only to see the numbers on the scale go up. No way! Instead of worrying about the scale, judge your progress by—most importantly—how you feel, and as for changes in your body, you can always take some initial measurements and then re-measure once a week. What has always worked best for me is simply to gauge how my clothes fit. That's the biggest tell of all. I have a pair of jean shorts I'm wearing right now. A couple of months ago I couldn't get them to even think about zipping! That's the only kind of progress I need. To me, numbers on the scale don't mean a whole lot.

Chapter Six: On Your Diet

It wouldn't be right to talk about gaining muscle and losing fat without talking a bit about diet.

I'm not going to go overboard but there are a few things I'd like to touch on.

First off, as I previously spoke about at the end of chapter four—the scale—I forgot to mention another reason I don't care to use them. Most of them have a tendency to fluctuate as much as five pounds in less than twenty-four hours. In other words, if I'm going by the scale, I often will have "gained" five pounds from when I got up to when it's time for bed.

Not cool.

Not possible, either. Our bodies are made up of an estimated sixty-five percent water. It is normal for the amount of water in our bodies to fluctuate all the time. Losing water weight does not equate to losing fat. However, while we are trying to lose weight, and while we're working out, it is especially important to keep our bodies hydrated.

There are as many theories on the web as you could click on about how much water to drink, but for questions like these, I like to refer to the Mayo Clinic website, because I know that the information they put out there has been thoroughly researched. What follows is their advice on water intake:

Every single day, you lose water by breathing, sweating, urinating, and pooping. To function properly, your body's water must be replenished through the consumption of food and beverages.

The average healthy man who lives in a temperate climate needs 15.5 cups or 3.7 liters of fluids every day, and the average healthy woman living in the same place needs 11.5 cups or 2.7 liters every day.

This is about what I do for myself in a normal day and it seems to work. Regardless, don't skimp on the water.

There's another important factor when it comes to building muscle and that is protein. If you are serious about adding some muscle mass, you're going to need to eat your protein. That doesn't mean it has to be meat; there are plenty of non-meat options for protein intake. Of course, if you are a vegetarian you already know that.

Another little tip: your body needs fat to lose fat. Sounds strange, doesn't it? But if your body is starved of nutrients, it will begin to hold on to everything it has instinctually, and as a result, you won't see any weight loss.

There are a million types of "diets" out there, and this is not a book about diets so I'm not going to delve into them. If I were going to say anything at all about your diet (and don't get me wrong, your diet IS important,) I would say two words: eat clean.

What does that mean? Since clean is the opposite of dirty, in this case, think dirty equals "processed."

Do your body a giant favor and stay away from processed foods! Eat foods that are as "close" to the earth as you can.

- Lean proteins (including fish and non-meat proteins)
- Tons—and I do really mean tons—of vegetables
- Lean fat (avocado, almonds, coconut oil)
- Dairy (full-fat; eat sparingly)
- Fruits (sparingly)

It's that simple. No "TV Dinners." No boxes of macaroni and cheese, please. Nothing that has a "bunch" of ingredients, many of which you aren't even familiar with. Those are bad. Leave them in the store.

If you have a sweet tooth, indulge it, but rarely, and even a sweet tooth can be indulged in a healthy manner. There's nothing wrong with eating some strawberries topped with full fat whipped cream. Yummy!

Well, there you have it. You really are set. Everything is explained and condensed for you.

Start your weight training and your cardio, eat clean, drink your water and reap the rewards.

Go get 'em!

PART V

Chapter 1: Meal Planning 101

Sticking to a diet is something that is not the easiest in the world. When it comes down to it, we struggle to change up our diets on a whim. It might be that for the first few days, you are able to stick to it and make sure that you are only eating those foods that are better for you, but over time, you will get to a point where you feel the pressure to cave in. You might realize that sticking to your diet is difficult and think that stopping for a burger on your way home won't be too bad. You might think that figuring out lunch or dinner is too much of a hassle, or you realize that the foods that you have bought forgot a key ingredient that you needed for dinner.

The good news is, you have an easy fix. When you are able to figure out what you are making for yourself for your meals well in advance, you stop having to worry so much about the foods that you eat, what you do with them, and what you are going to reach for when it's time to eat. You will be able to change up what you are doing so that you can be certain that the meals that you are enjoying are good for you, and you won't have to worry so much about the stress that goes into it. Let's take a look at what you need to do to get started with meal planning so that you can begin to do so without having to think too much about it.

Make a Menu

First, before you do anything, make sure that you make a menu! This should be something that you do on your own, or you should sit down with your family to ask them what they prefer. If you can do this, you will be able to ensure that you've got a clear-cut plan. When you have a menu a week in advance, you save yourself time and money because you know that all of your meals will use ingredients that are similar, and you won't have to spend forever thinking about what you should make at any point in time.

Plan around Ads

When you do your menu, make it a point to glance through the weekly ads as well. Typically, you will find that there are plenty of deals that you can make use of that will save you money.

Go Meatless Once Per Week

A great thing to do that is highly recommended on the Mediterranean Diet is to have a day each week where you go meatless for dinner. By doing so, you will realize that you can actually cut costs and enjoy the foods more at the same time. It is a great way to get that additional fruit and veggie content into your day, and there are plenty of healthy options that are out there for you. You just have to commit to doing so. In the meal plans that you'll see below, you will notice that there will be a meatless day on Day 2 every week.

Use Ingredients That You Already Have On Hand

Make it a point to use ingredients that you already have on hand whenever possible. Alternatively, make sure that all of the meals that you eat during the week use very similar ingredients. When you do this, you know that you're avoiding causing any waste or losing ingredients along the way, meaning that you can save money. The good news is, on the Mediterranean diet, there are plenty of delicious meals that enjoy very similar ingredients that you can eat.

Avoid Recipes that Call for a Special Ingredient

If you're trying to avoid waste, it is a good idea for you to avoid any ingredients in meals that are not going to carry over to other meals during your weekly plan. By avoiding doing so, you can usually save yourself that money for that one ingredient that would be wasted. Alternatively, if you find that you really want that dish, try seeing if you can freeze some of it for later. When you do that, you can usually ensure that your special ingredient at least didn't go to waste.

Use Seasonal Foods

Fruits and veggies are usually cheaper when you buy them in season, and even better, when you do so, you will be enjoying a basic factor of the Mediterranean diet just by virtue of enjoying the foods when they are fresh. Fresher foods are usually tastier, and they also tend to carry more vitamins and minerals because they have not had the chance to degrade over time.

Make Use of Leftovers and Extra Portions

One of the greatest things that you can do when it comes to meal planning is to make use of your leftovers and make-ahead meals. When you do this regularly, making larger portions than you need, you can then use the extras as lunches and dinners all week long, meaning that you won't have to be constantly worrying about the food that you eat for lunch. We will use some of these in the meal plans that you will see as well.

Eat What You Enjoy

Finally, the last thing to remember with your meal plan is that you ought to be enjoying the foods that are on it at all times. When you ensure that the foods that you have on your plate are those that you actually enjoy, sticking to your meal plan doesn't become such a chore, and that means that you will be able to do better as well with your own diet. Your meal plan should be loaded up with foods that you are actually excited about enjoying. Meal planning and dieting should not be a drag—you should love every moment of it!

Chapter 2: 1 Month Meal Plan

This meal plan is designed to be used for one month to help you simplify making sure that you have delicious meals to eat without having to think. These meals are fantastic options if you don't know where to start but want to enjoy your Mediterranean diet without much hassle. For each of the five weeks included, you will get one breakfast recipe, one lunch recipe, one dinner recipe, and one snack recipe to make meal planning a breeze. So, give these recipes a try! Many of them are so delicious, you'll want to enjoy them over and over again!

Week 1: Success is no accident—you have to reach for it

Mediterranean Breakfast Sandwich

Serves: 4

Time: 20 minutes

Ingredients:

- Baby spinach (2 c.)

- Eggs (4)

- Fresh rosemary (1 Tbsp.)

- Low-fat feta cheese (4 Tbsp.)

- Multigrain sandwich thins (4)

- Olive oil (4 tsp.)

- Salt and pepper according to preference

- Tomato (1, cut into 8 slices)

Instructions:

1. Preheat your oven. This recipe works best at 375° F. Cut the sandwich things in half and brush the insides with half of your olive oil. Place the things on a baking sheet and toast for about five minutes or until the edges are lightly browned and crispy.

2. In a large skillet, heat the rest of your olive oil and the rosemary. Use medium-high heat. Crack your eggs into the skillet one at a time. Cook until the whites have set while keeping the yolks runny. Break the yolks and flip the eggs until done.

3. Serve by placing spinach in between two sandwich thins, along with two tomato slices, an egg, and a tablespoon of feta cheese.

Greek Chicken Bowls

Serves: 4

Time: 20 minutes

Ingredients:

- Arugula (4 c.)
- Chicken breast tenders (1 lb.)

- Cucumber (1, diced)
- Curry powder (1 Tbsp.)
- Dried basil (1 tsp.)
- Garlic powder (1 tsp.)
- Kalamata olives (2 Tbsp.)
- Olive oil (1 Tbsp.)
- Pistachios (0.25 c., chopped)
- Red onion (half, sliced)
- Sunflower seeds (0.25 c.)
- Tzatziki sauce (1 c.)

Instructions:

1. In a bowl, mix in the chicken tenders, curry powder, dried basil, and garlic powder. Make sure to coat the chicken evenly.
2. Heat one tablespoon of olive oil over medium-high. Add the chicken and cook for about four minutes on each side. Remove from the pan and set aside to cool.
3. Place one cup of arugula into four bowls. Toss in the diced cucumber, onion, and kalamata olives.
4. Chop the chicken and distribute evenly between the four bowls.
5. Top with tzatziki sauce, pistachio seeds, and sunflower seeds.

Ratatouille

Serves: 8

Time: 1 hour 30 minutes

Ingredients:

- Crushed tomatoes (1 28 oz. can)
- Eggplants (2)
- Fresh basil (4 Tbsp., chopped)
- Fresh parsley (2 Tbsp., chopped)
- Fresh thyme (2 tsp.)
- Garlic cloves (4, minced and 1 tsp, minced)
- Olive oil (6 Tbsp.)
- Onion (1, diced)
- Red bell pepper (1, diced)
- Roma tomatoes (6)
- Salt and pepper to personal preference
- Yellow bell pepper (1, diced)
- Yellow squashes (2)
- Zucchinis (2)

Instructions:

1. Get your oven ready. This recipe works best at 375° F.
2. Slice the tomatoes, eggplant, squash, and zucchini into thin rounds and set them to the side.

3. Heat up two tablespoons of olive oil in an oven safe pan using medium-high heat. Sauté your onions, four cloves of garlic, and bell peppers for about ten minutes or when soft. Add in your pepper and salt along with the full can of crushed tomatoes. Add in two tablespoons of basil. Stir thoroughly.

4. Take the vegetable slices from earlier and arrange them on top of the sauce in a pattern of your choosing. For example, a slice of eggplant, followed by a slice of tomato, squash, and zucchini, then repeating. Start from the outside and work inward to the center of your pan. Sprinkle salt and pepper overtop the veggies.

5. In a bowl, toss in the remaining basil and garlic, thyme, parsley, salt, pepper, and the rest of the olive oil. Mix it all together, and spoon over the veggies.

6. Cover your pan and bake for 40 minutes. Uncover and then continue baking for another 20 minutes.

Snack Platter

Serves: 6

Time:

Ingredients:

Rosemary Almonds

- Butter (1 Tbsp.)

- Dried rosemary (2 tsp.)
- Salt (pinch)
- Whole almonds (2 c.)

Hummus

- Chickpeas (1 15 oz. can, drained and rinsed)
- Garlic clove (1, peeled)
- Lemon (half, juiced)
- Olive oil (2 Tbsp.)
- Salt and pepper according to personal preference
- Tahini (2 Tbsp.)
- Water (2 Tbsp.)

Other sides

- Bell pepper (1, sliced)
- Cucumber (1, sliced)
- Feta cheese (4 oz, cubed)
- Kalamata olives (handful, drained)
- Pepperoncini peppers (6, drained)
- Pitas (6, sliced into wedges)
- Small fresh mozzarella balls (18)
- Soppressata (6 oz.)
- Sweet cherry peppers (18)

Instructions:

1. To get started, make your rosemary almonds. Take a large skillet and place it on a burner set to medium heat. Start melting the butter in, then toss in the almonds, rosemary and a bit of salt. Toss the nuts on occasion to ensure even coating.

2. Cook the almonds for roughly ten minutes, getting them nicely toasted. Set the almonds off to the side to let them cool.

3. Now you'll set out to make the hummus. Take a blender or food processor and toss in the hummus ingredients. Blend until you get a nice, smooth paste. If you find that your paste is too thick, try blending in a bit of water until you get the desired consistency. Once you have the right consistency, taste for seasoning and adjust as necessary.

4. Pour and scrape the hummus into a bowl and drizzle in a bit of olive oil. Set it off to the side to get the rest of the platter going.

5. Grab the sweet cherry peppers and stuff them with the little balls of mozzarella. Arrange a platter in any pattern you like. If serving for a party or family, try keeping each snack in its own little segment to keep things looking neat.

Week 2: Self-belief and effort will take you to what you want to achieve

Breakfast Quesadilla

Serves: 1

Time: 10 minutes

Ingredients:

- Basil (handful)
- Eggs (2)
- Flour tortilla (1)

- Green pesto (1 tsp.)
- Mozzarella (0.25 c.)
- Salt and pepper according to personal preference
- Tomato (half, sliced)

Instructions:

1. Scramble your eggs until just a little runny. Remember, you will be cooking them further inside the quesadilla. Season with salt and pepper.
2. Take the eggs and spread over half of the tortilla.
3. Add basil, pesto, mozzarella cheese, and the slices of tomato.
4. Fold your tortilla and toast on an oiled pan. Toast until both sides are golden brown.

Greek Orzo Salad

Serves: 6

Time: 25 minutes

Ingredients:

- Canned chickpeas (1 c., drained and rinsed)
- Dijon mustard (0.5 tsp)
- Dill (0.33 c., chopped)
- Dried oregano (1 tsp)
- English cucumber (half, diced)
- Feta cheese crumbles (0.5 c.)
- Kalamata olives (0.33 c., halved)
- Lemon (half, juice and zest)
- Mint (0.33 c., chopped)
- Olive oil (3 Tbsp.)
- Orzo pasta (1.25 c. when dry)
- Roasted red pepper (half, diced)
- Salt and pepper to taste
- Shallot (0.25 c., minced)
- White wine vinegar (2 Tbsp.)

Instructions:

1. Prepare the orzo according to the packaging details. Once the orzo is al dente, drain it and rinse until it drops to room temperature.
2. In a bowl, toss all the ingredients together until thoroughly incorporated.

One Pot Mediterranean Chicken

Serves: 4

Time: 1 hour

Ingredients:

- Chicken broth (3 c.)
- Chicken thighs (3, bone in, skin on)

- Chickpeas (1 15 oz can, drained and rinsed)
- Dried oregano (0.5 tsp.)
- Fresh parsley (2 Tbsp., chopped)
- Garlic cloves (2, minced)
- Kalamata olives (0.75 c., halved)
- Olive oil (2 tsp.)
- Onion (1, finely diced)
- Orzo pasta (8 ounces uncooked)
- Roasted peppers (0.5 c., chopped)
- Salt and pepper according to personal preference

Instructions:

1. Prepare your oven at 375°. Heat your olive oil in a large skillet over medium-high heat.
2. Season the chicken with salt and pepper on both sides. Toss the chicken into the skillet and cook for five minutes on each side, or until golden in color. Remove the chicken.
3. Take the skillet and drain most of the rendered fat, leaving about a teaspoon. Add the onion and cook for five minutes. Toss in the garlic and cook for an additional minute.
4. Now you will want to add the orzo, roasted peppers, oregano, chickpeas, and olives into the pan. Add in salt and pepper.
5. Place the thighs on top of the orzo and pour in the chicken broth.
6. Bring to a boil, then cover and place in the oven. Bake for 35 minutes or until chicken has cooked through. Top with parsley and serve.

Mediterranean Nachos

Serves: 6

Time: 10 minutes

Ingredients:

- Canned artichoke hearts (1 c., rinsed, drained, and dried)
- Canned garbanzo beans (0.75 c., rinsed, drained, and dried)
- Feta cheese (0.5 c., crumbled)
- Fresh cilantro (2 Tbsp., chopped)
- Pine nuts (2.5 Tbsp.)
- Roasted red peppers (0.5 c., dried)
- Sabra Hummus (half of their 10 oz. container)
- Tomatoes (0.5 c., chopped)
- Tortilla chips (roughly half a bag)

Instructions:

1. Get your oven ready by setting it to 375°F. In a baking pan, layer the tortilla chips, and spread hummus over them evenly. Top with garbanzo beans, red peppers, artichoke hearts, feta cheese, and pine nuts.
2. Bake for about five minutes or until warmed through. Remove the baking pan and top the nachos with fresh cilantro and tomatoes. Serve and enjoy.

Week 3: The harder you work, the greater the success

Breakfast Tostadas

Serves: 4

Time: 15 minutes

Ingredients:

- Beaten eggs (8)
- Cucumber (0.5 c., seeded and chopped)
- Feta (0.25 c., crumbled)
- Garlic powder (0.5 tsp)
- Green onions (0.5 c., chopped)
- Oregano (0.5 tsp)
- Red Pepper (0.5 c., diced)
- Roasted red pepper hummus (0.5 c.)
- Skim milk (0.5 c.)
- Tomatoes (0.5 c., diced)
- Tostadas (4)

Instructions:

1. In a large skillet, cook the red pepper for two minutes on medium heat until softened. Toss in the eggs, garlic powder, milk, oregano, and green onions. Stir constantly until the egg whites have set.
2. Top the tostadas with hummus, egg mixture, cucumber, feta, and tomatoes.

Roasted Vegetable Bowl

Serves: 2

Time: 45 minutes

Ingredients:

- Crushed red pepper flakes (a pinch)
- Fresh parsley (1 Tbsp., chopped)
- Kalamata olives (0.25 c.)
- Kale (1 c., ribboned)
- Lemon juice (1 Tbsp.)
- Marinated artichoke hearts (0.25 c., drained and chopped)
- Nutritional yeast (1 Tbsp.)
- Olive oil (1 Tbsp., then enough to drizzle)
- Salt and pepper to taste

- Spaghetti squash (half, seeds removed)
- Sun-dried tomatoes (2 Tbsp., chopped)
- Walnuts (0.25 c., chopped)

Instructions:

1. Get your oven ready by setting it to 400° F. Take a baking sheet and blanket it with parchment paper.

2. Take the squash half and place it on the parchment paper. Drizzle olive oil over the side that is cut, and season with salt and pepper. Turn it over so it is facing cut side down and bake for 40 minutes. It is ready when it is soft.

3. Remove the squash shell, and season with a bit more salt and pepper.

4. Stack the kale, artichoke hearts, walnuts, sun-dried tomatoes, and kalamata olives on the squash.

5. Squeeze the lemon juice over and drizzle olive oil. Finish with chopped parsley and a bit of crushed red pepper flakes.

Mediterranean Chicken

Serves: 4

Time: 40 minutes

Ingredients:

- Chicken breasts (1 lb., boneless, skinless)
- Chives (2 Tbsp., chopped)
- Feta cheese (0.25 c., crumbled)
- Garlic (1 tsp., minced)
- Italian seasoning (1 tsp.)
- Lemon juice (2 Tbsp.)
- Olive oil (2 Tbsp., and 1 Tbsp.)
- Salt and pepper according to personal preference
- Tomatoes (1 c., diced)

Instructions:

1. Pour in two tablespoons of olive oil, the lemon juice, salt, pepper, garlic, and Italian seasoning in a resealable plastic bag. Add in the chicken, seal and shake to coat the chicken.
2. Allow the chicken to marinate for at least 30 minutes in the refrigerator.
3. Heat the rest of the olive oil in a pan over medium heat.
4. Place the chicken on the pan and cook for five minutes on each side, or until cooked through.
5. In a bowl, mix the tomatoes, chives, and feta cheese. Season with salt and pepper.
6. When serving, spoon the tomato mixture on top of the chicken.

Baked Phyllo Chips

Serves: 2

Time: 10 minutes

Ingredients:

- Grated cheese (your choice)
- Olive oil (enough to brush with)
- Phyllo sheets (4)
- Salt and pepper according to personal preference

Instructions:

1. Get your oven ready by setting it to 350° F. Brush olive oil over a phyllo sheet generously. Sprinkle grated cheese and your seasoning on top.
2. Grab a second sheet of your phyllo and place it on top of the first one. Again, brush with olive oil and sprinkle cheese and seasoning on top.
3. Repeat this process with the remaining sheets of phyllo. Top the stack with cheese and seasoning.
4. Once complete, cut the stack of phyllo into bite-sized rectangles. A pizza cutter may be helpful here.
5. Grab a baking sheet and blanket it with some parchment paper. Take your phyllo rectangles and place them on the parchment paper.
6. Bake in the oven for about seven minutes or until they reach a golden color.
7. Remove them from the oven and allow them to cool before serving.

Week 4: You don't need perfection—you need effort

Mini Omelets

Serves: 8

Time: 40 minutes

Ingredients:

- Cheddar cheese (0.25 c., shredded)
- Eggs (8)
- Half and half (0.5 c.)
- Olive oil (2 tsps.)
- Salt and pepper according to personal preference
- Spinach (1 c., chopped)

Instructions:

1. Get your oven ready by setting it to 350° F. Prepare a muffin pan or ramekins by greasing them with olive oil.
2. In a bowl, beat the eggs and dairy until you have a fluffy consistency.
3. Stir in the cheese and your seasonings. Pour in the spinach and continue beating the eggs.
4. Pour the egg mixture into your ramekins or muffin pan.
5. Bake the omelets until they have set, which should be roughly 25 minutes. Remove them from the oven and allow them to cool before serving.

Basil Shrimp Salad

Serves: 2

Time: 40 minutes

Ingredients:

- Dried basil (1 tsp.)
- Lemon juice (1 Tbsp.)
- Olive oil (1 tsp.)
- Romaine lettuce (2 c.)
- Shrimp (12 medium or 8 large)
- White wine vinegar (0.25 c.)

Instructions:

1. Whisk together the white wine vinegar, olive oil, lemon juice, and basil. Stick your shrimp in the marinade for half an hour.

2. Take the marinade and shrimp and cook in a skillet over medium heat until cooked through.

3. Allow the shrimp to cool along with the juice and pour into a bowl. Toss in the romaine lettuce and mix well to get the flavor thoroughly infused in the salad. Serve.

Mediterranean Flounder

Serves: 4

Time: 40 minutes

Ingredients:

- Capers (0.25 c.)
- Diced tomatoes (1 can)
- Flounder fillets (1 lb.)
- Fresh basil (12 leaves, chopped)
- Fresh parmesan cheese (3 Tbsp., grated)
- Garlic cloves (2, chopped)
- Italian seasoning (a pinch)
- Kalamata olives (0.5 c., pitted and chopped)
- Lemon juice (1 tsp.)

- Red onion (half, chopped)
- White wine (0.25 c.)

Instructions:

1. Set your oven to 425° F. Take a skillet and pour in enough olive oil to sauté the onion until soft. Cook on medium-high heat.
2. Toss in the garlic, Italian seasoning, and tomatoes. Cook for an additional five minutes.
3. Pour in the wine, capers, olives, lemon juice, and only half of the basil you chopped.
4. Reduce the heat to low and stir in the parmesan cheese. Simmer for ten minutes or until the sauce has thickened.
5. Place the flounder fillets in a baking pan and pour the sauce over top. Sprinkle the remaining basil on top and bake for 12 minutes.

Nutty Energy Bites

Serves: 10

Time: 10 minutes

Ingredients:

- Dried dates (1 c., pitted)
- Almonds (0.5 c.)

- Pine nuts (0.25 c.)
- Flaxseeds (1 Tbsp., milled) Porridge oats (2 Tbsp.)
- Pistachios (0.25 c., coarsely ground)

Instructions:

1. Take the dates, pine nuts, milled flaxseeds, almonds, and porridge oats and pour them into a food processor or blender. Mix until thoroughly incorporated.
2. Using a tablespoon, scoop the mixture and roll it between your hands until you have a small, bite-sized ball. Do this until you have used the entirety of the dough. This recipe should be enough for about ten.
3. On a plate, sprinkle your ground pistachios. Take the energy balls and roll them on the pistachio grounds, making sure to coat them evenly. Serve or store in the refrigerator.

Week 5: Transformation Happens One Day at a Time

Mediterranean Breakfast Bowl

Serves: 1

Time: 25 minutes

Ingredients:

- Artichoke hearts (0.25 c., chopped)
- Baby arugula (2 c.)
- Capers (1 Tbsp.)
- Egg (1)
- Feta (2 Tbsp., crumbled)
- Garlic (0.25 tsp)
- Kalamata olives (5, chopped)
- Lemon thyme (1 Tbsp., chopped)
- Olive oil (0.5 Tbsp.)
- Pepper (0.25 tsp)
- Sun-dried tomatoes (2 Tbsp., chopped)
- Sweet potato (1 c., cubed)

Instructions:

1. Take your olive oil and, when hot, pan fry your sweet potatoes for 5-10 minutes until they have softened. Then, sprinkle on the seasonings.
2. Place arugula into a bowl, then top with potatoes, then everything but the egg.
3. Prepare the egg to your liking and serve.

Chicken Shawarma Pita Pockets

Serves: 6

Time: 40 minutes

Ingredients:

- Cayenne (0.5 tsp)
- Chicken thighs (8, boneless, skinless, bite-sized pieces)
- Cloves (0.5 tsp, ground)
- Garlic powder (0.75 Tbsp.)
- Ground cumin (0.75 Tbsp.)
- Lemon juice (1 lemon)
- Olive oil (0.33 c.)
- Onion (1, sliced thinly)
- Paprika (0.75 Tbsp.)
- Salt
- Turmeric powder (0.75 Tbsp.)

To serve:

- Pita pockets (6)
- Tzatziki sauce
- Arugula
- Diced tomatoes
- Diced onions
- Sliced Kalamata olives

Instructions:

1. Combine all spices. Then, place all chicken, already diced, into the bowl. Coat well, then toss in onions, lemon juice, and oil. Mix well and let marinade for at least 3 hours, or overnight.
2. Preheat the oven to 425 F. Allow chicken to sit at room temperature a few minutes. Then, spread it on an oiled sheet pan. Roast for 30 minutes.
3. To serve, fill up a pita pocket with tzatziki, chicken, arugula, and any toppings you prefer. Enjoy.

Turkey Mediterranean Casserole

Serves: 6

Time: 35 minutes

Ingredients:

- Fusilli pasta (0.5 lbs.)
- Turkey (1.5 c., chopped)
- Sun dried tomatoes (2 Tbsp., drained)
- Canned artichokes (7 oz., drained)
- Kalamata olives (3.5 oz., drained and chopped)
- Parsley (0.5 Tbsp., chopped and fresh)
- Basil (1 T, fresh)
- Salt and pepper to taste
- Marinara sauce (1 c.)

- Black chopped olives (2 oz., drained)
- Mozzarella cheese (1.5 c., shredded)

Instructions:

1. Warm your oven to 350 F. Prepare your pasta according to the directions, drain, and place into a bowl. Prepare your basil, parsley, olives, tomatoes, artichokes, and other ingredients.

2. Mix together the pasta with the turkey, tomatoes, olives, artichokes, herbs, seasoning, and marinara sauce. Give it a good mix to incorporate all of the ingredients evenly.

3. Take a 9x13 oven-safe dish and layer in the first half of your pasta mixture. Then, sprinkle on half of your mozzarella cheese. Top with the rest of the pasta, then sprinkle on the chopped black olives as well. Spread the rest of the shredded cheese on top, then bake it for 20-25 minutes. It is done when the cheese is all bubbly and the casserole is hot.

Heirloom Tomato and Cucumber Toast

Serves: 2

Time: 5 minutes

Ingredients:

- Heirloom tomato (1, diced)
- Persian cucumber (1, diced)
- Extra virgin olive oil (1 tsp)
- Oregano (a pinch, dried)
- Kosher salt and pepper
- Whipped cream cheese (2 tsp)
- Whole grain bread (2 pieces)
- Balsamic glaze (1 tsp)

Instructions:

4. Combine the tomato, cucumber, oil, and all seasonings together.
5. Spread cheese across bread, then top with mixture, followed by balsamic glaze.

Chapter 3: Maintaining Your Diet

Sticking to a diet can be tough. You could see that other people are having some great food and wish that you could enjoy it too. You might realize that you miss the foods that you used to eat and feel like it's a drag to not be able to enjoy them. When you are able to enjoy the foods that you are eating, sticking to your diet is far easier. However, that doesn't mean that you won't miss those old foods sometimes. Thankfully, the Mediterranean diet is not a very restrictive one—you are able to enjoy foods in moderation that would otherwise not be allowed, and because of that, you can take the slice of cake at the work party, or you can choose to pick up a coffee for yourself every now and then. When you do this, you're not doing anything wrong, so long as you enjoy food in moderation.

Within this chapter, we are going to take a look at several tips that you can use that will help you with maintaining your diet so that you will be able to stick to it, even when you feel like things are getting difficult. Think of this as your guide to avoiding giving in entirely—this will help you to do the best thing for yourself so that you can know that you are healthy. Now, let's get started.

Find Your Motivation

First, if you want to keep yourself on your diet, one of the best things that you can do is make sure that you find and stick to your motivation. Make sure that you know what it is in life that is motivating you. Are you losing weight because a doctor told you to? Fair enough—but how do you make that personal and about yourself? Maybe instead of looking at it as a purely health-related choice, look at it as something that you are doing because of yourself. Maybe you are eating better so that you are able to watch your children graduate or so that you can run after them at the park and stay healthy, even when it is hard to do so.

Remind Yourself Why You are Eating Healthily

When you find that you are struggling to eat healthily, remind yourself of why you are doing it in the first place. When you do this enough, you will begin to resist the urges easier than ever. Make it a point to tell yourself not to eat something a certain way. Take the time to remind yourself that you don't need to order that greasy pizza—you are eating better foods because you want to be there for your children or grandchildren.

Reminding yourself of your motivation is a great way to overcome those cravings that you may have at any point in time. The cravings that you have are usually strong and compelling, but if you learn to overcome them, you realize that they weren't actually as powerful as you thought they were. Defeat the cravings. Learn to tell yourself that they are not actually able to control you. Tell yourself that you can do better with yourself.

Eat Slowly

Now, on the Mediterranean diet, you should already be eating your meals with other people anyway. You should be taking the time to enjoy those meals while talking to other people and ensuring that you get that connection with them, and in doing so, you realize that you are able to do better. You realize that you are able to keep yourself under control longer, and that is a great way to defend and protect yourself from overeating.

When you eat slowly, you can get the same effect. Eating slowly means that you will have longer for your brain to realize that you should be eating less. When you are able to trigger that sensation of satiety because you were eating slowly, you end up eating fewer calories by default, and that matters immensely.

Keep Yourself Accountable

Don't forget that, ultimately, your diet is something that you must control on your own. Keep yourself accountable by making sure that you show other people what you are doing. If you are trying to lose weight, let them know, and tell them how you plan to do so. When you do this, you are able to remind yourself that other people know what you are doing and why—this is a great way to foster that sense of accountability because you will feel like you have to actually follow through, or you will be embarrassed by having to admit fault. You could also make accountability to yourself as well. When you do this, you are able to remind yourself that your diet is your own. Using apps to track your food and caloric intake is just one way that you can do this.

Remember Your Moderation

While it can be difficult to face a diet where you feel like you can't actually enjoy the foods that you would like to eat, the truth is that on the Mediterranean diet, you are totally okay to eat those foods that you like or miss if you do so in moderation. There is nothing that is absolutely forbidden on the Mediterranean diet—there are just foods that you should be restricting regularly. However, that doesn't mean that you can't have a treat every now and then.

Remembering to live in moderation will help you from feeling like you have to cheat or give up as well. When you are able to enjoy your diet and still enjoy the times where you want to enjoy your treats, you realize that there is actually a happy medium between sticking to the diet and deciding to quit entirely.

Identify the Difference between Hunger and Craving

Another great way to help yourself stick to your diet is to recognize that there is a very real difference between actually being hungry and just craving something to eat. In general, cravings are felt in the mouth—when you feel like you are salivating or like you need to eat something, but it is entirely in your head and mouth, you know that you have a craving. When you are truly hungry, you feel an emptiness in your stomach—you are able to know because your abdomen is where the motivation is coming from.

Being able to tell when you have a craving and when you are genuinely hungry, you can usually avoid eating extra calories that you didn't actually need. This is major—if you don't want to overeat, you need to know when your body actually needs something and when it just wants something. And if you find that you just want something, that's okay too—just find a way to move on from it. If you want to indulge a bit here and there, there's no harm in that!

Stick to the Meal Plan

When it comes to sticking to a diet, one of the easiest and most straightforward ways to do so is to just stick to your meal plan that you set up. You have it there for a reason—it is there for you to fall back on, and the sooner that you are willing to accept that, recognizing that ultimately, you can stay on track when you don't have to think about things too much, the better you will do. You will be able to succeed on your diet because you will know that you have those tools in place to protect you—they will be lined up to ensure that your diet is able to provide you with everything that you need and they will also be there so that you can know that you are on the right track.

Drink Plenty of Water

Another key to keeping yourself on track with your diet is to make sure that you drink plenty of water throughout the day. Oftentimes, we mistake our thirst with hunger and eat instead. Of course, if you're thirsty, food isn't going to really fix your problem, and you will end up continuing to mix up the sensation as you try to move past it. The more you eat, the thirstier you will get until you realize that you're full but still feeling "hungry." By drinking plenty of water any time that you think that you might want to eat, you will be able to keep yourself hydrated, and in addition, you will prevent yourself from unintentionally eating too much.

Eat Several Times Per Day

One of the best ways to keep yourself on track with your diet is to make sure that you are regularly eating. By eating throughout the day, making sure that you keep yourself full, it is easier to keep yourself strong enough to resist giving in to cravings or anything else. When you do this regularly, you will discover that you can actually keep away much of your cravings so that you are more successful in managing your diet.

Eating several times per day often involves small meals and snacks if you prefer to do so. Some people don't like doing this, but if you find that you're one of those people who will do well on a diet when you are never actually hungry enough to get desperate enough to break it, you will probably be just fine.

Fill Up on Protein

Another great way to protect yourself from giving in and caving on your diet is to make sure that you fill up on protein. Whether it comes from an animal or plant source, make sure that every time you eat, you have some sort of tangible protein source. This is the best way to keep yourself on track because protein keeps you fuller for longer. When you eat something that's loaded up with protein, you don't feel the need to eat as much later on. The protein is usually very dense, and that means that you get to resist feeling hungry for longer than you thought that you would.

Some easy proteins come from nuts—but make sure that you are mindful that you do not end up overeating during this process—you might unintentionally end up eating too many without realizing it. While you should be eating proteins regularly, make sure that you are mindful of calorie content as well!

Keep Only Healthy Foods

A common mistake that people make while dieting is that they end up caving when they realize that their home is filled up with foods that they shouldn't be eating. Perhaps you are the only person in your home that is attempting to diet. In this case, you may end up running into a situation where you have all sorts of non-compliant foods on hand. You might have chips for your kids or snacks that your partner likes to eat on hand. You may feel like it is difficult for you to stay firm when you have that to consider, and that means that you end up stuck in temptation.

One of the best ways to prevent this is to either cut all of the unhealthy junk out of your home entirely or make sure that you keep the off-limits foods in specific places so that you don't have to look at it and see it tempting you every time that you go to get a snack for yourself. By trying to keep yourself limited to just healthy foods, you will be healthier, and you will make better decisions.

Eat Breakfast Daily

Finally, make sure that breakfast is non-negotiable. Make sure that you enjoy it every single day, even if you're busy. This is where those make-ahead meals can come in handy; by knowing that you have to keep to a meal plan and knowing that you already have the food on hand, you can keep yourself fed. Breakfast sets you up for success or failure—if you want to truly succeed on your diet, you must make sure that you are willing to eat those healthier foods as much as possible, and you must get started on the right foot. Enjoy those foods first thing every day. Eat so that you are not ravenous when you finally do decide that it is time to sit down and find something to eat. Even if you just have a smoothie or something quick to eat as you go, having breakfast will help you to persevere.

PART VI

Vegetarian Cookbook

The vegetarian diet has gained immense popularity in the last few years. According to some studies, it has been found that an estimated 18% of the world population is vegetarian. Apart from all the environmental and ethical benefits of removing meat from the diet, a properly planned vegetarian diet can reduce the risk of various chronic diseases, improve diet quality, and help in losing weight. The vegetarian diet also does not include poultry and fish. The majority of the people opt for a vegetarian diet for personal or religious reasons and for ethical reasons, such as animal rights. Other people opt for it for various environmental reasons, like livestock production, which results in the emission of greenhouse gases.

A vegetarian diet comes along with a wide array of benefits. It has been found that vegetarians have a better quality of diet when compared to meat-eaters. They also have a higher intake of beneficial nutrients, such as vitamin C, fiber, magnesium, and vitamin E. Switching from a normal meat diet to a vegetarian diet can result to be an effective strategy in case you want to lose weight. For instance, in a review of twelve studies, it has been found that vegetarians can lose about four pounds of weight over eighteen weeks than non-vegetarians. Also, vegetarians have lower BMI or body mass index than non-vegetarians.

Some research found that a vegetarian diet can be linked to a lower risk of developing cancer and those of the colon, breast, stomach, and rectum. However, it lacks enough evidence to prove that a vegetarian diet can effectively reduce cancer risk. People who follow a vegetarian diet can maintain healthy levels of blood sugar. It can also help in preventing the onset of diabetes by controlling the levels of blood sugar. Vegetarian diets help in the reduction of various heart diseases that can make your heart stronger and healthier.

A vegetarian diet needs to include a wide mixture of veggies, fruits, healthy fats, grains, and proteins. To replace the protein that you get from meat in a diet, you will need to include plant foods rich in proteins such as seeds, nuts, legumes, seitan, tofu, and tempeh. Consuming whole foods rich in nutrients, such as vegetables and fruits, can provide your body with the necessary minerals and vitamins to fill the nutritional gaps in a diet. Some of the food items that you can include in your diet are:

- **Fruits:** Bananas, apples, melons, oranges, peaches, pears

- **Vegetables:** Asparagus, leafy greens, carrots, broccoli

- **Legumes:** Beans, lentils, chickpeas, peas

- **Seeds:** Chia, flaxseed, hemp

- **Nuts:** Walnuts, cashews, almonds

- **Proteins:** Seitan, natto, tofu, eggs, tempeh

You cannot include food items such as fish, seafood, meat, poultry, and ingredients that are based on meat. Restriction of eggs and dairy products are applicable for the vegans and not for vegetarians. I have included some tasty and easy vegetarian recipes that will help you to plan your diet effectively.

Chapter 1: Breakfast Recipes

No matter which diet you follow, breakfast is very important in all cases. In this section, you will find some easy-to-make and tasty breakfast recipes that you can include in your vegetarian diet.

Black Bean Bowl

Total Prep & Cooking Time: Fifteen minutes

Yields: Two servings

Nutrition Facts: Calories: 620.1 | Protein: 28.9g | Carbs: 47.6g | Fat: 37.1g | Fiber: 23.2g

Ingredients:

- Two tbsps. of olive oil

- Four eggs (beaten)
- One can of black beans (rinsed)
- One avocado (sliced)
- One-fourth cup of salsa
- One tsp. of each
  - Black pepper (ground)
  - Salt

Method:

1. Take a small pan and heat oil in it. Add the eggs and scramble for five minutes.

2. Place the beans in a bowl. Heat the beans in the oven for one minute.

3. Divide the beans into two serving bowls.

4. Top the beans with scrambled eggs, salsa, and avocado. Add pepper and salt according to taste.

Coconut Blueberry Ricotta Bowl

Total Prep & Cooking Time: Twenty minutes

Yields: One serving

Nutrition Facts: Calories: 303.2 | Protein: 9.5g | Carbs: 32.1g | Fat: 15.3g | Fiber: 3.9g

Ingredients:

- One-fourth cup of ricotta cheese
- One tbsp. of each
    - Honey
    - Coconut milk
    - Slivered almonds
    - Coconut flakes
- Half cup of blueberries

Method:

1. Combine coconut milk and ricotta in a medium-sized bowl. Drizzle honey from the top and add coconut and almonds.

2. Serve with blueberries from the top.

Broccoli Quiche

Total Prep & Cooking Time: Fifty minutes

Yields: Six servings

Nutrition Facts: Calories: 378.2 | Protein: 17.3g | Carbs: 21.1g | Fat: 25.8g | Fiber: 3.1g

Ingredients:

- One pie crust (unbaked)
- Three tbsps. of butter
- One onion (minced)
- One tsp. of each
  - Garlic (minced)
  - Salt
- Two cups of broccoli (chopped)
- One and a half cup of mozzarella cheese (shredded)
- Four eggs (beaten)
- Two and a half cup of milk
- Half tsp. of black pepper
- One tbsp. of butter (melted)

Method

;

1. Start by preheating your oven at 175 degrees Celsius. Use pie crust for lining a deep pie pan.

2. Take a large saucepan and add butter to it. Add broccoli, onion, and garlic. Cook the veggies slowly until tender. Add the cooked veggies to the pie crust and add cheese from the top.

3. Mix milk and eggs in a bowl; add pepper and salt for seasoning. Add the remaining butter to the milk mixture. Pour the mixture over the mixture of vegetables.

4. Bake the quiche in the oven for forty minutes or until the center has properly set.

Tomato Bagel Sandwich

Total Prep & Cooking Time: Twenty minutes

Yields: One serving

Nutrition Facts: Calories: 346.3 | Protein: 13.1g | Carbs: 48.6g | Fat: 10.7g | Fiber: 2.9g

Ingredients:

- One bagel (split, toasted)
- Two tbsps. of cream cheese
- One large tomato (sliced thinly)
- Pepper and salt (to season)
- Four basil leaves

Method:

1. Spread the cream cheese on the halves of the bagel.

2. Top the cheese layer with slices of tomato. Add pepper and salt for seasoning.

3. Serve with basil leaves from the top.

Cornmeal And Blueberry Pancakes

Total Prep & Cooking Time: Thirty minutes

Yields: Six servings

Nutrition Facts: Calories: 180.3 | Protein: 5.2g | Carbs: 26.8g | Fat: 5.1g | Fiber: 4.6g

Ingredients:

- One cup of soy milk
- Half cup of each
  - Water
  - Cornmeal (ground)
- One and a half cup of wheat flour
- One tsp. baking powder
- One-third tsp. baking soda
- One-fourth tsp. of salt
- One cup of blueberries
- Two tbsps. of vegetable oil

Method:

1. Preheat your oven at 95 degrees Celsius.

2. Combine water and soy milk in a bowl.

3. Take a large mixing bowl and combine cornmeal, baking soda, flour, salt, and baking powder. Add the mixture of soy milk. Combine properly. Add the blueberries and allow the batter to rest for five minutes.

4. Take a large skillet and grease it using oil. Add one-fourth cup of the batter in the skillet. Cook until the pancakes are bubbly on the top, and the edges are dry. Cook for five minutes on each side. Repeat with the remaining batter.

5. Serve hot with jam or syrup.

Breakfast Tortilla

Total Prep & Cooking Time: Twenty minutes

Yields: Two servings

Nutrition Facts: Calories: 381.3 | Protein: 15.8g | Carbs: 38.1g | Fat: 18.7g | Fiber: 4.5g

Ingredients:

- Two tbsps. of beans (refried)
- Three tbsps. of salsa
- Three large eggs (beaten)
- One tbsp. of mayonnaise
- Four tortillas (flour)
- One and a half cup of lettuce (shredded)

Method:

1. Combine salsa and beans in a small bowl.

2. Take an iron skillet and heat oil in it. Add the eggs and let the bottom set—Cook for one minute. Spread the mixture of beans on half of the egg and flip one side for making the shape of a half-circle. Cook until the eggs set properly.

3. Spread mayonnaise on the tortillas.

4. Cut the cooked eggs into four equal pieces. Place each piece of eggs on the tortillas. Top with lettuce.

5. Roll the tortillas. Serve hot.

Zucchini Frittata

Total Prep & Cooking Time: Forty minutes

Yields: Five servings

Nutrition Facts: Calories: 258.3 | Protein: 14.2g | Carbs: 9.1g | Fat: 19.6g | Fiber: 3.4g

Ingredients:

- One cup of water
- Three tbsps. of olive oil
- Half tsp. of salt
- Half bell pepper (green, chopped)
- Three zucchinis (cut in slices of half-inch)
- Two garlic cloves (peeled)
- One onion (diced)
- Six mushrooms (chopped)
- One tbsp. of butter
- Five eggs
- Pepper and salt (to taste)
- One and a half cup of mozzarella cheese (shredded)
- Three tbsps. of parmesan cheese

Method:

1. Start by preheating your oven at 160/175 degrees Celsius.

2. Take a large skillet and combine olive oil, water, green pepper, salt, garlic cloves, and zucchini. Simmer the mixture until the zucchini is soft— Cook for seven minutes.

3. Drain the water and remove the garlic; add mushroom, onion, and butter. Keep cooking until the onion turns transparent. Add the eggs and keep stirring. Add pepper and salt for seasoning. Cook until the eggs are firm.

4. Add mozzarella cheese from the top.

5. Bake in the oven for ten minutes.

6. Remove the frittata from the oven and add parmesan cheese from the top. Place under the broiler for about five minutes.

7. Cut the frittata in wedges and serve warm.

Oatmeal And Strawberry Smoothie

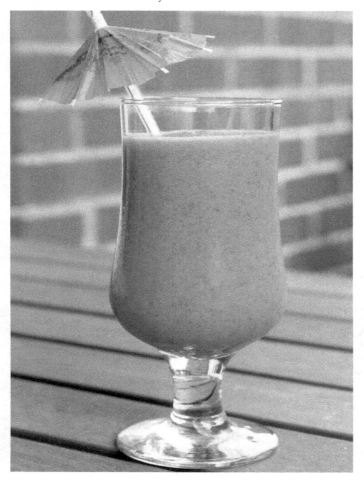

Total Prep & Cooking Time: Twenty minutes

Yields: Two servings

Nutrition Facts: Calories: 204.1 | Protein: 5.2g | Carbs: 41.3g | Fat: 2.7g | Fiber: 6.9g

Ingredients:

- One cup of almond milk
- Half cup of rolled oats
- Fourteen strawberries (frozen)
- One banana (cut in chunks)
- Two tsps. of agave nectar
- Half tsp. of vanilla extract

Method:

1. Add almond milk, strawberries, oats, agave nectar, banana, and vanilla extract in a food processor. Keep blending until smooth.

2. Serve with pieces of strawberry from the top.

Chapter 2: Appetizers Recipes

Hosting a party but not sure which appetizers to prepare as most of your guests are vegetarians? No worries as I have included some great vegetarian recipes for appetizers in this section.

Buffalo Cauliflower

Total Prep & Cooking Time: Thirty minutes

Yields: Twelve servings

Nutrition Facts: Calories: 120 | Protein: 4.2g | Carbs: 7.9g | Fat: 8.7g | Fiber: 2.3g

Ingredients:

- One serving of cooking spray
- Half cup of buffalo sauce
- Three tbsps. of mayonnaise
- One large egg
- Six cups of cauliflower florets
- Two cups of garlic croutons
- One-fourth cup of parmesan cheese (grated)

For the dipping sauce:

- One-fourth cup of each
  - Sour cream
  - Blue cheese salad dressing
- One tsp. of black pepper (ground)

Method:

1. Start by preheating your oven to 230 degrees Celsius. Use a cooking spray for greasing a baking tray.

2. Combine mayonnaise, buffalo sauce, and egg in a bowl. Toss the florets of cauliflower in the mixture of sauce and coat properly.

3. Spread the tossed florets on the baking tray.

4. Add the croutons on a blender and pulse them into crumbs. Add the cheese and pulse again. Spread the mixture of cheese and croutons over the florets of cauliflower.

5. Bake for fifteen minutes until tender and browned. Allow the florets to sit for five minutes.

6. Mix all the ingredients for the dipping sauce.

7. Serve cauliflower florets with dip sauce by the side.

Garlic Bread And Veggie Delight

Total Prep & Cooking Time: Thirty minutes

Yields: Five servings

Nutrition Facts: Calories: 390.2 | Protein: 12.4g | Carbs: 58.7g | Fat: 11.6g | Fiber: 7.2g

Ingredients:

- One cup of olive oil
- One garlic clove (chopped)
- One eggplant (cubed)
- One zucchini (cubed)
- One tomato (chopped)
- One tsp. of salt
- Two tsps. of each
  - Basil (minced)
  - Oregano (minced)
- One baguette
- Four tsps. of garlic powder
- Six tsps. of butter

Method:

1. Take a large skillet and add olive oil to it. Add garlic and fry for two minutes until browned.

2. Add the zucchini and eggplant to the skillet and cook for five minutes. Make sure that the eggplant is tender and brown.

3. Add the chunks of tomato and combine the veggies; add basil, oregano, and salt. Cook for two minutes and remove from heat.

4. Preheat oven 140/165 degrees Celsius.

5. Slice the baguette into one-inch slices, approximately twelve slices. Add butter and garlic powder on the bread slices and place them on the oven rack. Heat the bread for five minutes.

6. Arrange the heated bread slices on a plate. Top the slices with vegetables.

7. Serve immediately.

Spinach Parmesan Balls

Total Prep & Cooking Time: Thirty minutes

Yields: Ten servings

Nutrition Facts: Calories: 254.1 | Protein: 11.4g | Carbs: 18.4g | Fat: 14.2g | Fiber: 3.5g

Ingredients:

- Twenty ounces of frozen spinach (chopped)
- Two cups of bread crumbs
- One cup of parmesan cheese (grated)
- Half cup of butter (melted)
- Four green onions (chopped)
- Four eggs (beaten)
- Pepper and salt (for seasoning)

Method:

1. Start by preheating your oven at 175 degrees Celsius.

2. Take a bowl and combine spinach, bread crumbs, cheese, green onions, butter, pepper, salt, and eggs. Make balls of one-inch size from the prepared mixture.

3. Arrange the spinach balls on a baking tray. Bake for fifteen minutes until browned.

4. Serve hot.

Cheese Garlic Bread

Total Prep & Cooking Time: Thirty minutes

Yields: Eight servings

Nutrition Facts: Calories: 260 | Protein: 7.1g | Carbs: 29.7g | Fat: 11.4g | Fiber: 1.5g

Ingredients:

- Half cup of butter (melted)
- One tsp. of garlic salt
- One-fourth tsp. of rosemary (dried)
- One-eighth tsp. of each
  - Basil (dried)
  - Thyme (dried)
  - Garlic powder
- One tbsp. of parmesan cheese (grated)
- One loaf of French bread (halved)

Method:

1. Preheat oven at 150 degrees Celsius.

2. Mix garlic salt, butter, basil, rosemary, thyme, garlic powder, and cheese in a bowl.

3. Spread the butter mixture on the halves of the bread. Add extra cheese from the top if you want to.

4. Place halves of bread on a baking tray. Bake for twelve minutes until browned.

Stuffed Mushrooms

Total Prep & Cooking Time: Forty-five minutes

Yields: Twelve servings

Nutrition Facts: Calories: 89 | Protein: 2.6g | Carbs: 1.3g | Fat: 8.9g | Fiber: 0.6g

Ingredients:

- Twelve whole mushrooms
- One tbsp. of each
    - Minced garlic
    - Vegetable oil
- Eight ounces of cream cheese (softened)
- One-fourth cup of parmesan cheese (grated)
- One-fourth tsp. of each
    - Onion powder
    - Black pepper (ground)
    - Cayenne powder (ground)

Method:

1. Preheat the oven to 175 degrees Celsius. Grease a baking tray with the help of cooking spray.

2. Clean the mushrooms using a damp kitchen towel; break the stems. Chop the mushroom stems finely.

3. Take a skillet and heat oil in it. Add chopped stems of mushroom and garlic—Cook for five minutes.

4. Remove the skillet from heat and let it cool. Add the cream cheese, black pepper, parmesan cheese, cayenne powder, and onion powder. Mix well.

5. Use a small spoon for filling the mushroom caps with the mushroom stuffing.

6. Place the mushroom caps on the prepared baking tray.

7. Bake for twenty minutes until liquid forms under the mushroom caps.

Tomato Bruschetta

Total Prep & Cooking Time: Thirty-five minutes

Yields: Twelve servings

Nutrition Facts: Calories: 214.1 | Protein: 10.6g | Carbs: 23.1g | Fat: 8.8g | Fiber: 2.6g

Ingredients:

- Six tomatoes (chopped)
- Half cup of sun-dried tomatoes
- Three garlic cloves (minced)
- One-fourth cup of olive oil
- Two tbsps. of balsamic vinegar
- One-third cup of basil
- One-fourth tsp. of each
  - Black pepper (ground)
  - Salt
- One baguette
- Two cups of mozzarella cheese (shredded)

Method:

1. Preheat your oven on the setting of broiler.

2. Combine tomatoes, olive oil, vinegar, garlic, sun-dried tomatoes, basil, pepper, and salt in a bowl. Let the mixture sit for ten minutes.

3. Cut the baguette into slices of a three-fourth inch. Arrange the baguette slices on a baking tray. Broil for two minutes until browned.

4. Add the mixture of tomatoes on the slices of bread and top with mozzarella cheese.

5. Broil again for five minutes.

Spicy Pumpkin Seeds

Total Prep & Cooking Time: One hour and ten minutes

Yields: Eight servings

Nutrition Facts: Calories: 91 | Protein: 3.2g | Carbs: 8.8g | Fat: 4.9g | Fiber: 0.7g

Ingredients:

- Two tbsps. of margarine
- Half tsp. of salt
- One-eighth tsp. of garlic salt
- Two tsps. of Worcestershire sauce
- Two cups of pumpkin seeds (raw)

Method:

1. Preheat your oven at 135 degrees Celsius.

2. Combine the ingredients in a mixing bowl.

3. Bake for one hour. Stir in between.

Chapter 3: Soups & Side Dishes Recipes

Soup forms an integral part of a vegetarian diet along with the side dishes. Here are some easy vegetarian recipes for side dishes and soups that you can include in your diet.

Carrot Soup

Total Prep & Cooking Time: Forty-five minutes

Yields: Four servings

Nutrition Facts: Calories: 351 | Protein: 3.2g | Carbs: 23.1g | Fat: 29.7g | Fiber: 4.2g

Ingredients:

- Two tbsps. of olive oil
- Four-hundred grams of carrots (cut in disks of half-inch)
- Half onion (diced)
- Four cloves of garlic (smashed)
- Two tsps. of cumin seeds
- Four cups of vegetable stock
- Two bay leaves
- One tsp. of salt
- One-fourth tsp. of white pepper
- Two tsps. of honey
- One-fourth cup of yogurt

Method:

1. Take a heavy bottom pan and add oil in it. Add onions, garlic, and cumin to the pan. Sauté on a medium flame for six minutes until tender and golden in color. Stir occasionally.

2. Add the stock, carrots, salt, bay leaves, white pepper, and simmer the mixture. Cover the pan and simmer for twenty minutes. Allow the soup to cool down for five minutes.

3. Use an immersion blender for blending the soup. Blend until you reach a silky smooth consistency.

4. Return the soup to heat and add honey. Stir the soup. Add yogurt and simmer. Taste the soup and adjust the seasonings. Keep the soup warm on very low flame until you serve.

5. Divide the soup among serving bowls. Serve with a dollop of yogurt from the top.

Note: You can use ground spices in place of the whole spices. But, whole spices will help in adding extra flavor.

Celery Soup

Total Prep & Cooking Time: Thirty-five minutes

Yields: Seven servings

Nutrition Facts: Calories: 180 | Protein: 4.2g | Carbs: 23.1g | Fat: 9.2g | Fiber: 4.9g

Ingredients:

- Two tbsps. of olive oil
- One onion (diced)
- Four cloves of garlic (chopped)
- Six cups of celery (thinly sliced)
- Two cups of potatoes (sliced in rounds)
- Four cups of vegetable stock

- One cup of water
- One bay leaf
- One tsp. of salt
- Half tsp. of pepper
- One-third tsp. of cayenne
- Half cup of sour cream
- One-fourth cup of each
    - Parsley (small stems)
    - Dill (small stems)

Method:

1. Take a large pot and add oil in it. Heat the oil and start adding the onion. Cook for five minutes until golden.

2. Roughly chop celery, potatoes, and garlic. Add garlic and cook the mixture for two minutes. Add potatoes, celery, stock, bay leaf, water, salt, cayenne, and pepper. The liquid needs to be enough to cover the vegetables. Cover the pot and boil the mixture. Simmer for ten minutes.

3. Remove bay leaf after turning off the stove. Add herbs to the pot and allow them to wilt.

4. Take an immersion blender and start blending the soup until silky smooth.

5. Return the pot to heat and cook over low flame for five minutes.

6. Serve with sour cream from the top.

Tomato Soup And Halloumi Croutons

Total Prep & Cooking Time: One hour and five minutes

Yields: Six servings

Nutrition Facts: Calories: 285 | Protein: 10.3g | Carbs: 13.2g | Fat: 23.2g | Fiber: 4.9g

Ingredients:

- Three pounds of tomatoes
- Half red onion (sliced in thin rings)
- Six cloves of garlic
- Two tsps. of thyme leaves

- One-third cup of oil
- Four cups of vegetable stock
- One-fourth cup of basil leaves (chopped)
- One cup of Greek yogurt

For croutons:

- One block of halloumi cheese (cut in cubes of three-fourth inch)
- One tbsp. of oil

Method:

1. Start by preheating your oven at 200 degrees Celsius.

2. Use parchment paper for lining baking sheet. Spread the onions, tomatoes, and garlic on the sheet. Drizzle with some oil from the top—roast in the oven for thirty minutes.

3. Heat some oil in a pan and start adding the halloumi cubes. Cook for four minutes until golden on all sides.

4. Add the roasted veggies in a pot along with the vegetable stock. Use an immersion blender for blending the soup until smooth. Place the pot over a low flame and add seasonings of your choice. Simmer the soup and add basil. Simmer for ten minutes.

5. Add half a cup of yogurt to the soup.

6. Serve the soup in serving bowls with croutons from the top.

Baked Potatoes And Mushrooms With Spinach

Total Prep & Cooking Time: Forty-five minutes

Yields: Four servings

Nutrition Facts: Calories: 235.1 | Protein: 7.1g | Carbs: 27.1g | Fat: 11.3g | Fiber: 4.9g

Ingredients:

- One pound of potatoes (halved)
- Three tbsps. of olive oil
- Half pound of Portobello mushroom
- Six garlic cloves
- Two tbsps. of thyme (chopped)
- One pinch of black pepper and salt
- One-fourth cup of cherry tomatoes
- Half cup of spinach (sliced)
- Two tbsps. of pine nuts (toasted)

Method:

1. Preheat your oven at 200/220 degrees Celsius.

2. Add the potatoes in a roasting pan and drizzle some oil from the top. Roast the potatoes for fifteen minutes.

3. Add mushrooms along with garlic to the pan. Add thyme from the top along with some olive oil. Sprinkle black pepper and salt. Roast again for five minutes.

4. Add cherry tomatoes to the pan. Cook again for five minutes until the mushrooms are tender.

5. Add toasted pine nuts from the top and serve with spinach by the side.

Garlic Potatoes

Total Prep & Cooking Time: Fifty minutes

Yields: Four servings

Nutrition Facts: Calories: 270.2 | Protein: 5.2g | Carbs: 39.7g | Fat: 12.1g | Fiber: 4.9g

Ingredients:

- Two pounds of red potatoes (quartered)
- One-fourth cup of butter (melted)
- Two tsps. of garlic (minced)
- One tsp. of salt
- One lemon (juiced)
- One tbsp. of parmesan cheese (grated)

Method:

1. Start by preheating the oven at 175 degrees Celsius.

2. Place the potatoes in a baking dish.

3. Combine butter, lemon juice, garlic, and salt in a small bowl. Add this mixture over the potatoes and stir for coating. Add parmesan cheese from the top.

4. Bake the potatoes by covering the dish in the preheated oven for thirty minutes. Remove the cover and bake again for ten minutes.

Buttery Carrots

Total Prep & Cooking Time: Twenty-five minutes

Yields: Four servings

Nutrition Facts: Calories: 182.3 | Protein: 0.8g | Carbs: 21.3g | Fat: 10.3g | Fiber: 3.9g

Ingredients:

- One pound of baby carrots
- One-fourth cup of margarine
- One-third cup of brown sugar

Method:

1. Cook the baby carrots in boiling water. Drain most of the liquid leaving behind a little bit of liquid at the base.

2. Remove the carrots from the pot. Add brown sugar along with margarine. Simmer the mixture for two minutes and add the carrots to the pot. Toss well for combining.

3. Serve warm.

Chapter 4: Main Course Recipes

After you are done with the soups and side dishes, now it is time to jump into the main course. Here are some tasty main course recipes that you can include within your vegetarian diet plan.

Nut And Tofu Loaf

Total Prep & Cooking Time: One hour and forty minutes

Yields: Six servings

Nutrition Facts: Calories: 308.3 | Protein: 15.2g | Carbs: 27.6g | Fat: 14.2g | Fiber: 4.8g

Ingredients:

- One serving of cooking spray
- Twelve ounces of tofu (firm, drained, cubed)
- Two large eggs
- One ounce dry mix of onion soup
- One tbsp. of soy sauce
- Three-fourth cup of walnuts (chopped)
- One tsp. of olive oil
- Eight ounces of fresh mushrooms (sliced)
- One onion (chopped)
- Two celery stalks (chopped)
- Two tsps. of oregano (dried)
- One and a half tsps. of basil (dried)
- Half tsp. of sage (dried)
- Two cups of bread crumbs

Method:

1. Start by preheating the oven at 175 degrees Celsius. Use a cooking spray for greasing loaf pan.

2. Place eggs, tofu, soy sauce, and onion soup mix in a blender. Blend the ingredients until properly combined. Add the walnuts and blend again. Transfer the mixture of tofu to a bowl.

3. Take a large skillet and heat oil in it. Add mushrooms and cook them for four minutes. Add celery and cook for two minutes—season with basil, sage, and oregano.

4. Stir bread crumbs and veggies into the mixture of tofu. Press the loaf mixture into the pan.

5. Bake the loaf in the oven for sixty to seventy minutes.

6. Let the loaf cool down for five minutes before serving.

7. Slice the loaf and serve warm.

Velvety Chickpea Curry

Total Prep & Cooking Time: Forty-five minutes

Yields: Six servings

Nutrition Facts: Calories: 408.3 | Protein: 10.2g | Carbs: 68.3g | Fat: 11.2g | Fiber: 8.9g

Ingredients:

- One tbsp. of each
  - Ginger root (minced)
  - Coconut oil
- One onion (sliced)
- Four garlic cloves (minced)
- Two tbsps. of curry powder
- One-fourth tsp. of pepper flakes
- Three cups of vegetable stock
- Two tbsps. of each
  - Soy sauce
  - Tomato paste
  - Maple syrup
- Half pound of potatoes (cut in pieces of a three-fourth inch)
- One carrot (sliced)
- Four cups of cauliflower florets
- One can of chickpeas (rinsed)
- Half cup of coconut milk
- One-fourth cup of cilantro (chopped)
- Half cup of peas (frozen)
- Salt (for seasoning)

Method:

1. Take a heavy-based pot and melt coconut oil in it. Add onions to the pot and sauté for five minutes. Add garlic and ginger to the pot—Cook for thirty seconds. Add pepper flakes, curry powder, soy sauce, stock, tomato paste, and maple syrup. Stir well.

2. Add carrots and potatoes to the pot and cover. Boil the mixture. Slightly open the cover and simmer for ten minutes. Add chickpeas, cauliflower, cilantro, and coconut milk. Stir well for combining. Simmer again for seven minutes. Add peas and cook for one minute.

3. Season with salt and cook for one minute.

4. Serve with basmati rice and cilantro from the top.

Tofu Pad Thai

Total Prep & Cooking Time: Forty-five minutes

Yields: Four servings

Nutrition Facts: Calories: 451 | Protein: 15.4g | Carbs: 60.1g | Fat: 15.2g | Fiber: 4.2g

Ingredients:

- Twelve ounces of tofu (drained, cubed)
- One tbsp. of cornstarch
- Three tbsps. of vegetable oil
- Eight ounces of rice noodles

For the sauce:

- One-fourth cup of each
  - Sriracha sauce
  - Water
  - Soy sauce
- Two tbsps. of white sugar
- One tbsp. of tamarind concentrate
- One tsp. of pepper flakes
- One large egg

- Two tbsps. of spring onions (chopped)
- One and a half tbsp. of peanuts (crushed)
- One lime (cut in wedges)

Method:

1. Coat the tofu cubes with cornstarch in a large bowl.

2. Heat two tbsps. of oil in a skillet. Fry the coated tofu for two minutes on each side.

3. Place the rice noodles in a medium bowl. Cover the noodles using hot boiling water. Soak the noodles until soft for three minutes. Drain the water.

4. Mix sriracha sauce, water, sugar, soy sauce, pepper flakes, and tamarind concentrate in a skillet. Cook for five minutes.

5. Heat one tbsp. of oil in a large wok. Add noodles, onion, along with the tofu. Cook the mixture for three minutes. Add sauce and toss it for combining.

6. Push the noodles to a side and crack the egg in the center. Stir for thirty seconds and mix with the noodles.

7. Serve with peanuts, green onion, and wedges of lime.

Eggplant Parmesan

Total Prep & Cooking Time: One hour

Yields: Ten servings

Nutrition Facts: Calories: 480.2 | Protein: 21.2g | Carbs: 60.1g | Fat: 15.2g | Fiber: 9.8g

Ingredients:

- Three eggplants (sliced)
- Two eggs (beaten)
- Four cups of bread crumbs
- Six cups of spaghetti sauce
- Sixteen ounces of mozzarella cheese (shredded)
- Half cup of parmesan cheese
- Half tsp. of basil (dried)

Method:

1. Preheat the oven at 175 degrees Celsius.

2. Dip the slices of eggplant in egg and then coat in bread crumbs.

3. Arrange the slices of eggplant in a baking sheet and bake for five minutes on both sides.

4. Take a baking dish and spread the spaghetti sauce for covering the base. Arrange the eggplant slices over the sauce. Sprinkle cheese from the top. Repeat for the remaining layers. Top with basil and cheese.

5. Bake for thirty-minutes until browned.

Veg Korma

Total Prep & Cooking Time: Fifty-five minutes

Yields: Four servings

Nutrition Facts: Calories: 451 | Protein: 8.4g | Carbs: 40.1g | Fat: 30.2g | Fiber: 8.7g

Ingredients:

- Two tbsps. of vegetable oil
- One onion (diced)
- One tsp. of ginger root (minced)
- Four garlic cloves (minced)
- Two potatoes (cubed)
- Four carrots (cubed)
- One jalapeno pepper (sliced)
- Three tbsps. of cashews (ground)
- One can of tomato sauce
- Two tsps. of salt
- One and a half tbsps. of curry powder
- One cup of green peas (frozen)
- One red bell pepper (roughly chopped)
- One-third yellow bell pepper (roughly chopped)
- One bunch of cilantro
- Half cup of heavy cream

Method:

1. Take a skillet and heat oil in it. Add onions to the oil and cook until soft. Add garlic and ginger to the skillet. Cook for one minute. Add carrots, potatoes, cashews, jalapenos, and tomato sauce. Add curry powder and season with salt. Stir well and cook for ten minutes until the potatoes are soft.

2. Add bell pepper, peas, and cream. Lower the flame and cover the skillet—Cook for ten minutes.

3. Serve with cilantro from the top.

Mac And Cheese

Total Prep & Cooking Time: Fifty minutes

Yields: Six servings

Nutrition Facts: Calories: 456 | Protein: 24g | Carbs: 33.1g | Fat: 24.9g | Fiber: 2.3g

Ingredients:

- Two cups of elbow macaroni (uncooked)
- One-fourth cup of butter
- Two tbsps. of flour
- One tsp. of each
  - Black pepper (ground)
  - Mustard powder
- Two cups of milk
- Eight ounces of each
  - Cheese food (cubed)
  - American cheese (cubed)
- Half cup of bread crumbs

Method:

1. Preheat the oven at 180/200 degrees Celsius. Take a casserole dish and grease with butter.

2. Boil water in a pot with salt. Add the pasta and cook the pasta for six minutes. Drain the water.

3. Take a saucepan. Melt butter in it. Add mustard powder, flour, and pepper. Add milk and stir constantly. Add the cheeses and mix for two minutes until the sauce thickens.

4. Add the macaroni to the cheese mixture. Mix well.

5. Transfer the pasta mixture to the greased dish. Add bread crumbs from the top.

6. Bake for twenty minutes by covering the dish.

7. Serve hot.

Sesame Noodles

Total Prep & Cooking Time: Thirty minutes

Yields: Eight servings

Nutrition Facts: Calories: 365.2 | Protein: 7.3g | Carbs: 51.1g | Fat: 13.2g | Fiber: 3.9g

Ingredients:

- Sixteen ounces of linguine pasta
- Six garlic cloves (minced)
- Six tbsps. of each
    - Safflower oil
    - Sugar
    - Rice vinegar
    - Soy sauce
- Two tsps. of chili sauce
- Two tbsps. of sesame oil
- Six green onions (sliced)
- One tsp. of sesame seeds (toasted)

Method:

1. Boil water in a large pot along with some salt. Add the pasta. Keep cooking for eight minutes. Drain all the water.

2. Take a saucepan and heat oil in it. Add garlic, sugar, soy sauce, chili sauce, and sesame oil. Boil the mixture until the sugar gets dissolved.

3. Add the sauce to the cooked pasta and toss well for combining.

4. Serve with sesame seeds and green onions from the top.

Chapter 5: Dessert Recipes

Having a great dessert after a tasty meal can make you, as well as your stomach, feel good. So, here are some vegetarian dessert recipes for you.

Raspberry And Rosewater Sponge Cake

Total Prep & Cooking Time: Fifty-five minutes

Yields: Ten servings

Nutrition Facts: Calories: 441 | Protein: 4.1g | Carbs: 51.3g | Fat: 23.1g | Fiber: 1.3g

Ingredients:

- Two-hundred grams of butter (softened)
- Two-hundred and fifty grams of caster sugar
- Four eggs (beaten)
- One tsp. of vanilla extract
- Two cups of flour

For the rose filling:

- Half cup of double cream
- One tsp. of rosewater
- Four tbsps. of raspberry jam
- One-third cup of raspberries (crushed)

For rose icing:

- Half cup of icing sugar
- Half tsp. of rosewater

Method:

1. Heat the oven at 160 degrees Celsius.

2. Use parchment paper for lining two baking tins—grease with butter.

3. Mix sugar and butter in a bowl. Add the eggs and mix again.

4. Add vanilla extract to the egg mixture and mix. Add flour and fold.

5. Divide the cake batter into the prepared baking tins and bake in the oven for twenty minutes. Let the cakes cool for ten minutes.

6. Whisk double cream along with rosewater. Add the jam and mix.

7. Place one of the cakes on a serving plate and add the cream mixture. Add raspberries from the top and place the other cake on top.

8. Mix all the ingredients for the icing.

9. Serve the cake with rose icing from the top.

Easy Tiramisu

Total Prep & Cooking Time: One hour and fifteen minutes

Yields: Two servings

Nutrition Facts: Calories: 741 | Protein: 11.3g | Carbs: 44.3g | Fat: 51.6g | Fiber: 1.9g

Ingredients:

- Three tsps. of coffee granules
- Three tbsps. of coffee liqueur
- One and a half cup of mascarpone
- Half cup of condensed milk
- Six sponge fingers
- One tbsp. of cocoa powder

Method:

1. Mix coffee granules in two tbsps. of boiling water and stir for combining. Add three tbsps. of cold water along with coffee liqueur. Pour the mixture in a dish and keep aside.

2. Beat condensed milk, mascarpone, and vanilla extract in a bowl using a hand blender.

3. Break the fingers into two pieces and soak them in the mixture of coffee for thirty seconds.

4. Take a sundae glass and add the sponge fingers at the base. Add the cream mixture on top. Sift cocoa powder and chill in the refrigerator for one hour.

Chocolate Marquise

Total Prep & Cooking Time: Two hours and fifty-five minutes

Yields: Ten servings

Nutrition Facts: Calories: 710.3 | Protein: 7.8g | Carbs: 59.8g | Fat: 53g | Fiber: 1.5g

Ingredients:

- Three-hundred grams of dark chocolate
- Half cup of each
  - Caster sugar
  - Butter (softened)
- Six tbsps. of cocoa powder
- Six eggs
- One-third cup of double cream
- One-fourth cup of mint chocolate

Method:

1. Break the dark chocolate in small pieces and melt it using a double boiler system.

2. Beat butter and sugar in a bowl until creamy.

3. Separate the egg whites and yolks.

4. Mix the yolks with the sugar mixture until creamy.

5. Whip the double cream in another bowl.

6. Add the melted chocolate in the mixture of butter and fold gently. Add the whipped cream and mix well.

7. Spoon the mixture of chocolate in a piping bag.

8. Take a baking tin and pipe one layer of chocolate at the base of the tin. Cover the tin with pieces of mint chocolate. Repeat for the other layers. You will need to make four layers of mint chocolate.

9. Cover the tin with a cling film.

10. Chill the marquise in the fridge for two hours.

11. Remove the marquise from the tin by using a sharp knife.

12. Serve by cutting into slices.

Lemon Syllabub

Total Prep & Cooking Time: Fifteen minutes

Yields: Four servings

Nutrition Facts: Calories: 328 | Protein: 2.2g | Carbs: 14.6g | Fat: 28.6g | Fiber: 0.2g

Ingredients:

- Two cups of whipping cream
- Half cup of caster sugar
- Three tbsps. of white wine
- Half a lemon (juice and zest)
- Berries (for serving)

Method:

1. Mix sugar and whipping cream in a bowl. Whip until soft peaks are formed.

2. Add white wine in the mixture. Mix well. Add lemon juice and lemon zest in the mixture. Combine the ingredients properly.

3. Spoon the mixture into serving bowls or glasses.

4. Sprinkle remaining lemon zest from the top.

5. Serve the lemon syllabub with berries.

Note: You can use a mix of berries or only one type of berry.

CPSIA information can be obtained
at www.ICGtesting.com
Printed in the USA
LVHW051730070221
678648LV00020B/899

9 789814 950916